DIET AND HEALTH
═══IN═══
MODERN BRITAIN

EDITED BY
DEREK J. ODDY AND
DEREK S. MILLER

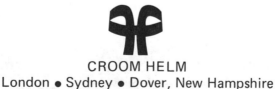

CROOM HELM
London • Sydney • Dover, New Hampshire

© 1985 Derek Oddy and Derek Miller
Croom Helm Ltd, Provident House, Burrell Row,
Beckenham, Kent BR3 1AT
Croom Helm Australia Pty Ltd, First Floor,
139 King Street, Sydney, NSW 2001, Australia

British Library Cataloguing in Publication Data

Diet and health in modern Britain.
   1. Diet—Great Britain—History—19th
   century. 2. Diet—Great Britain—History
   —20th century.
   I. Oddy, Derek J. II. Miller, Derek S.
   613.2'0941   RA784

   ISBN 0-7099-1922-0

Croom Helm, 51 Washington Street, Dover,
New Hampshire 03820, USA

Library of Congress Catalog in Publication Data
applied for.

Printed and bound in Great Britain by
Biddles Ltd, Guildford and King's Lynn

CONTENTS

List of Tables and Figures
Introduction   ... 1

1.   Colin Holmes   Science and practice ... 5
                         in arable farming
                         1910-1950

2.   Magnus Pyke   The impact of modern ... 32
                         food technology on
                         nutrition in the
                         twentieth century

3.   Richard Perren   The retail and whole-... 46
                         sale meat trade
                         1880-1939

4.   Forrest Capie   The demand for meat ... 66
                         in England and Wales
                         between the two World
                         Wars

5.   John Mark   Changes in the brew- ... 81
                         ing industry in the
                         twentieth century

6.   Peter Atkins   The production and   ...102
                         marketing of fruit
                         and vegetables
                         1850-1950

7.   Arnold Bender   The nutritional   ...134
                         importance of fruit
                         and vegetables

8.   Ian Buchanan   Infant feeding,   ...148
                           sanitation and
                           diarrhoea in colliery
                           communities
                           1880-1911

9.   John Hurt   Feeding the hungry   ...178
                           schoolchild in the
                           first half of the
                           twentieth century

10. Valerie Johnston   Local prison diets   ...207
                           1835-1878

11. Robert Thorne   The public house   ...231
                           reform movement

12. Dorothy   Rationing and   ...255
       Hollingsworth   economic constraints
                           on food consumption
                           since the Second
                           World War

13. Derek Miller   Man's demand for   ...274
                           energy

14. Pamela Mumford   The cost of nutrients...296
                           in the first half of
                           the twentieth
                           century

15. Alice Copping   The founding fathers   ...317
                           of the Nutrition
                           Society

Contributors 326

LIST OF TABLES AND FIGURES

Tables

1.1 Original network of state-financed research stations, 1911-14 6

1.2 Major additions to the original research
network, 1919-50 7

1.3 Estimated annual consumption of fertilizers 12

1.4 Farmers' annual average expenditure on
fertilizers 13

1.5 Farm draught power supplies, 1910-50 . 16

1.6 Farmers' expenditure on machinery ... 17

1.7 Yields per acre of main crops,1910-50 19

1.8 Acreage of main crops and temporary
pasture, 1910-50 22

1.9 Production of main crops, 1910-50 ... 24

1.10 Value of farm crops as a percentage of
value of gross agricultural output .. 25

1.11 Farmers' expenditure on selected
imputs, 1910-50 26

3.1 Annual average meat supply 48

4.1 A sample of the principal price, income
and substitution elasticities for meat
in the inter-war period 70

4.2 Meat consumption in different income
groups 76

5.1   The changing structure of the industry   82

5.2   Concentration ratios   82

5.3   Materials used in beer production   88

6.1   Quantities of home grown fruit and vegetables sold in London's markets 1851   116

6.2   Percentage of London's fruit and vegetables sold by Costermongers,1851....   119

6.3   London's fruit and vegetable Salesmen,
1817-50   120

6.4   Monthly revenue from Covent Garden 1870   123

6.5   Variability of demand for fruit and
vegetables with income   125

6.6   Regional demand for canned fruits and
vegetables, 1931-2   126

6.7   Comparison of the demand for fruit and
vegetables in London 1851 / 1978   127

7.1   Composition of vegetables   136

7.2   Contribution to the average intake of
nutrients from fruit and vegetables ..   140

7.3   Energy and protein content of fruit and
vegetables   144

8.1   Mortality from infant diarrhoea   152

8.2   Deaths per thousand live births   154

8.3   Methods of feeding infants   156

10.1   Recommended weekly diets for prisoners
1843   210

10.2   The 1878 system of classification   213

10.3   Variety of food in prison diets, 1850's   219

10.4   Daily nutrient intake of the Official
Dietaries, 1878   222

12.1   Percentage changes in the consumption of
certain foods during World War I & II   256

12.2   Food supplies after World War II   258

12.4   Comparison of weekly rations   263

12.5   Comparison of average weekly milk purchases
        1938-9 and 1943 265
13.1   Communities living on low food intakes   278
13.2   Daily energy requirements 280
13.3   Staple foods of the World 284
13.5   World food consumption 289
13.6   Food consumption in relation to production
        by area 290
13.7   Man's energy needs and land area 291
13.8   Retail cost of food in relation to intake 292
14.1   Annual yield of nutrients per acre 298
14.2   Cost of nutrients as purchased in different
        foods in London. March 1965 300
14.3   Survey of food prices, 1965-75 305
14.4   Cheapest energy sources 307
14.5   Cheapest protein sources 308
14.6   Cheapest calcium sources 309
14.7   Cheapest iron sources 310
14.8   Cheapest sources of vitamin A 311
14.9   Cheapest sources of vitamin C 312
14.10   Relative cost of energy 1890-1938 314
14.11   Relative cost of protein 1890-1938 315

Figures
1.1   Expenditure on the state research network   8
1.2   Estimated tractor numbers 1910-50   14
13.1   Energy intakes and gross national product 275
13.2   Population distribution 281
13.3   National diets of man 282
13.4   Regional diets of man 283
13.5   Primary and secondary human food prod-
        uction 289

INTRODUCTION

The appearance of a second volume of papers given at the Historians and Nutritionists Seminar at Queen Elizabeth College, University of London, reflects the success of the earlier collection which was published in 1976 as The Making of the Modern British Diet. The selection of papers gathered together in the present volume is in a similar vein to the earlier book, concentrating upon diet and health in Britain in the nineteenth and twentieth centuries.

Producing some coherence from the topics discussed at a seminar which is particularly wide-ranging in its interests and contributing disciplines, poses a problem for the editors. When The Making of the Modern British Diet reached the reviewers, one comment that interested us suggested that there was a need for more editorial guidance for readers. This led us to consider whether in this volume each paper or group of papers should be introduced by an editorial gloss. Although a case can be made out for such intervention, after some thought we have chosen to restrict our comments and give more space instead to the papers themselves. Unlike conference proceedings, papers given to a seminar at intervals are really too disparate to be linked in this way nor should the resulting collection of essays be confused with a textbook. Besides which, any editorial attempt to draw them together artificially would require so extensive an introduction that the papers' importance as research monographs would be reduced. Such a disclaimer of editorial responsibility is not intended to suggest that the seminar to which these papers have been given is an haphazard affair: there has been an underlying theme to the Seminar (on occasions implicit rather than obvious) over

1

the years when these papers were read to it. The chosen ground for the meeting of our separate disciplines was the examination of what goes on in a period of rapid social development. The work of nutritionists in the Third World causes them to ask historians, and social scientists in general for that matter, what happened in Britain? How did the problems of urban life in the nineteenth and early-twentieth centuries come to be solved? Britain had problems such as high infant and child mortality until the early part of the twentieth century: what caused this and how as it brought down? How did family life go on in conditions when income was low and sometimes intermittent, when protected water supplies and proper sanitation were not available, and when food preservation and food technology were still limited? How did the state devise diets for those in its care? What were the choices available for consumers?

To ask contributors to a seminar to have such a check-list in mind when writing their papers would daunt all but the most sanguine. We have never tried to pin our contributors down by such a frame of reference, though the interests of some members of our seminar do follow this line of inquiry. Possibly, indeed, the interface between different disciplines is the correct place to ask the questions which may otherwise be ignored. Few historians, other than mediaevalists in search of lost villages, don gumboots and engage in field-work: we hope the wider perspectives of this Seminar will stimulate historians to engage in metaphorical field-work at least; to see, for example, in the conditions of London and the industrial towns of nineteenth-century Britain some similarity to the open sewers of present-day Calcutta. Nutritionists facing such a situation in reality must tackle the problem before them with diagnostic techniques rather than detailed observation: similar techniques may also serve historians whose opportunities for empirical observation of past societies are limited to the preserved records of their existence. Conversely, there are lessons from history which it is essential for nutritionists to learn: past societies where poverty was the overriding factor have an obvious message for today. Within the last century problems of food production, distribution, and technology have all been overcome in Britain. The magnitude of these changes is such that, in present-day terms, they are as great as the contrast between North and South in the

Brandt Report. Such a comparison with present-day Third World problems may seem a false prospectus for a book in which only one paper deals directly with nutritional problems current in the contemporary world. What is demanded of the reader is the recognition that both the Britain of the late-nineteenth and early-twentieth centuries and life in the Third World today represent similar stages of the same process of demographic transition. Between the mid-nineteenth century and the outbreak of the Second World War, crude birth and death rates and the infant mortality rate (IMR) underwent major reductions in Britain. Over this period the birth rate fell from around 35 per thousand to less than 16, the death rate from around 20 per thousand to about 12, and the IMR from some 160 per thousand live births to about 60. Since these figures would serve as a rough approximation to the trends which have been developing over the last thirty years in the Third World, the connection would seem to be an important parallel, though the very marked slow-down in natural increase which occurred in Britain has not yet been replicated in the Third World.

Of course, the Seminar has had an interactive effect which has modified its general theme: its paradigm is in part at least the result of a self-generating process. On occasion, members of the Seminar have asked whether a paper could be arranged on a topic where there seems to be a gap in our knowledge; sometimes interest in one paper has led on to another - our papers on meat by Richard Perren and Forrest Capie, and on vegetables by Peter Atkins and Arnold Bender spring from such an interaction. Perhaps, also, we have been asking more sophisticated questions than we were earlier when The Making of the Modern British Diet represented our concern to know more about trends in supply and demand as the market for food developed in Britain during the period of industrialization. Certainly we have wanted to know more about the impact of science and technology on food production and the papers by Colin Holmes, Magnus Pyke, and John Mark arose for this reason. We have also asked questions about the changing presentation of food to consumers which has led us to discuss a range of topics from infant feeding to meals in schools and prisons and to examine the public house as a microcosm of behavioural change.

Some of our contributors may therefore have

3

been unconscious of their contribution in creating a paradigm within which the Seminar was operating and which led the Seminar's organizers to seek papers in a similar vein to those previously read to it. So much did this emerging process provide a rationale for our discussions that in 1978 we were able to convince the (then) Social Science Research Council that the Seminar deserved a modest level of financial support. We have been most grateful for that and the royalties from The Making of the Modern British Diet for keeping the Seminar going. The fact that our proceedings have always been enlivened by a buffet supper and some wine has been another form of field-work which all of us have enjoyed: such social occasions have often generated the better part of the discussion.

Publications arising from the Seminar

T. C. Barker, J.C. McKenzie, and John Yudkin, (eds.) Our Changing Fare (1966).

T. C. Barker, D.J. Oddy and John Yudkin, The Dietary Surveys of Dr. Edward Smith 1862-3 (1970).

T. C. Barker and John Yudkin (eds.) Fish in Britain (1971).

D. J. Oddy and D.S. Miller, (eds.) The Making of the Modern British Diet (1976).

1. SCIENCE AND PRACTICE IN ENGLISH ARABLE FARMING, 1910-1950(1)

C.J. HOLMES

Before 1910 the government was spending only a few hundred pounds each year(2) specifically on agricultural research. The Development and Road Improvement Fund Acts of 1909 and 1910 created a fund of £2,900,000 to be spent on selected aspects of rural economic development, and agricultural science was one of the designated activities(3). Thus central government became involved in the systematic, large-scale, financial support of agricultural research in Great Britain. An initial research network was established, based on eleven existing centres and one new one. All were in operation by the outbreak of the First World War in 1914. These first twelve centres are identified in Table 1.1 - the new creation was the Institute of Agricultural Economics at Oxford. Further expansion was halted by the outbreak of the first war and the ensuing need for financial stringency. However, if the immediate effect of the war was to retard the growth of the embryonic research network, its longer-term effect was the creation of a wider scheme than might otherwise have developed(4). In general, it soon became clear to agricultural experts just how much strength Germany was drawing from the support given to agricultural science there. Specifically, Britain's food production campaign of 1917 showed that strict control of quality in agricultural seeds and crops was a matter of urgent necessity. Also, the more widespread use of labour-saving machinery in wartime pointed to the need for a research institute in agricultural engineering. Accordingly, a National Institute of Agricultural Botany and two Plant Breeding Institutes were created in 1919, and in 1924 a centre for research in agricultural engineering was established(5).

Table 1.1: <u>Original network of state-financed research stations established 1911-1914
in England and Wales</u>

Subject	Centre
Plant Nutrition and Soil Science	Rothamsted
Plant Physiology	The Imperial College of Science and Technology
Plant Breeding	School of Agriculture, Cambridge University
Plant Breeding	The John Innes Institute for Horticulture
Plant Pathology	Kew, Royal Botanic Gardens
Animal Nutrition	Department of Genetics, Cambridge University
Dairy Science	University College, Reading
Helminthology	University of Birmingham
Entomology	University of Manchester
Agricultural Economics	Institute of Agricultural Economics, Oxford University
Animal Pathology	Royal Veterinary College, London
Fruit Husbandry	Wye College and Bristol University

Table 1.2 contains a list of the major research centres set up between 1919 and 1949.

Annual average expenditure on the state research network, hitherto unrecorded by agricultural economists or historians, amounted to £47,000
for 1911-14, £301,000 for 1931-34, rising to
£1,838,400 by 1947-50. The proportion coming from
non-government sources is estimated at 28 per cent
for 1911-14, 13 per cent for 1931-34, and 9 per
cent for 1947-50(6). In Figure 1.1 research expenditure is plotted in constant prices(7), to
take account of inflation. The sharp increase

Table 1.2: <u>Major additions to the original research</u>
<u>network in England and Wales 1919-50</u>

Subject	Year	Centre
Seed-testing and distribution	1919	National Institute of Agricultural Botany, University of Cambridge
Plant Breeding	1919	Plant Breeding Institute, University College of Wales, Aberystwyth
Plant Breeding	1919	Plant Breeding Institute, Cambridge University
Horticulture	1922	Horticultural Research Station, Cambridge University
Animal Breeding	1922	Animal Breeding Station, Department of Genetics, Cambridge University
Veterinary research	1923	Institute of Animal Pathology, Cambridge University
Poultry research	1923-5	National Poultry Institute Scheme, Harper Adams College, Wye College
Agricultural Engineering	1924	Institute of Agricultural Engineering, Oxford University, (re-located in Yorkshire in 1942)
Grassland research	1940	Grassland Research Station, Drayton, Bucks
Poultry Breeding	1948	Poultry Genetics Station, Cambridge University
Horticulture	1949	National Vegetable Research Station, Cambridge University

Figure 1.1

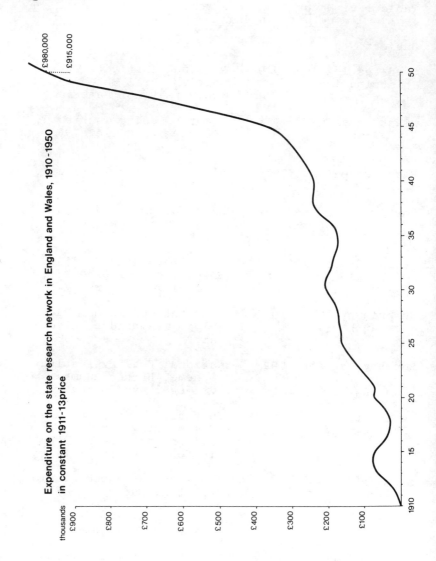

Expenditure on the state research network in England and Wales, 1910-1950 in constant 1911-13 price

Sources: see notes 8 and 9

in expenditure over the 1940s is evident, as is the retarding effect of the First World War. On the other hand, fiscal stringency in the early 1930s had a decidedly more adverse effect than the financial conditions prevailing in World War Two.

One of the greatest single scientific achievements for agriculture was the perfection of a process whereby ammonia could be produced from atmospheric nitrogen for use in fertilizers. The first men to achieve this were Birkeland and Eyde in Norway in 1905, but their process was only practical where electricity was cheap and plentiful. By 1909 Dr. Haber, in Germany, had perfected a better method for the fixation of atmospheric nitrogen. A mixture of nitrogen and hydrogen was heated under pressure and passed over a catalyst, calcium sulphate, the resultant gases combined to form ammonia gas ($N_2 + 3H_2 = 2NH_3$). Commercial production of ammonia was begun in Germany in 1913 (8). Nitrogen, of course, is used in the manufacture of explosives. By 1916 Britain was experiencing severe difficulties in obtaining her imported supply of natural nitrates from Chile, and the task of producing synthetic nitrates in this country assumed a new importance. Details of the Haber process were known, and the government decided to build a factory for the purpose at Billingham, County Durham. At the end of the war the factory was still being built, and the enterprise was passed over to Brunner, Mond and Company. Synthetic ammonia was first produced at Billingham on Christmas Eve, 1923.

Within the next decade there followed three important advances in fertilizer manufacture(9). In 1927 the Billingham factory produced a powdered fertilizer called 'Nitrochalk' - ammonium sulphate mixed with (insufficient(10)) quantities of beneficent lime. In 1929 'Nitrochalk' was produced in granular form, which made for ease of handling and application. Then, in 1931, a new range of fertilizers was introduced: complete, in that they contained all three of the basic plant foods, and concentrated, in that they had a much higher plant food content than conventional English fertilizer mixtures - 39 per cent as opposed to 13½ per cent. Brunner Mond, meanwhile, had combined with three other companies in 1926 to form Imperial Chemical Industries, and it must be said that I.C.I. played a leading part in the improvement of fertilizers and the advance of fertilizer research. The

9

company set up its own experimental station in
1928 and, from the start, Jealott's Hill won a
high reputation in the world of agricultural
science(11).

What did the state research network contribute
to the advance of fertilizer science? A great
number of field experiments produced an enormous
quantity of data which, by their very nature, could
be useful to farmers. At Rothamsted the statis-
tician Ronald Fisher established new statistical
techniques to interpret the results(12). When
analyzed, these experimental data revealed basic
differences in the effects of nitrates, phosphates
and potash on plant growth; they measured the response of different crops and varieties to fertilizer applications; they clarified the influence
of such factors as weather and soil conditions
on the action of fertilizers(13). In short, this
type of research showed farmers how to get the
best possible results from their fertilizers.

It seems that advances in farming practice
did not keep up with progress in fertilizer research. During the Second World War the War Agricultural Executive Committees found quite widespread ignorance amongst farmers on issues that
fertilizer specialists regarded as clear-cut.
Much newly ploughed pasture, for instance, was
found to be deficient in phosphates, and farmers
in traditional grassland areas were using far less
than the recommended doses of nitrates and pot-
ash(14). It has been said that neglect of field
drainage and the diminishing number of livestock
kept on arable farms minimized the effect of
fertilizers on crop yields(15). However, probably
the biggest single factor which limited the response of crops was a long-term decline in the
practice of regularly applying lime to the land.
As the use of artificials increased, the practice
of liming abated(16). Farmers clung to a widely
held but seriously mistaken belief that basic slag
and other chemical fertilizers sufficiently replaced lime lost naturally from the soil. The
reverse was known to be true: the cumulative effects
of superphosphate and the growing use of sulphate
of ammonia actually accelerated the rate of lime
loss. As early as 1921 it was estimated that only
44 per cent of lime lost from the soil each year
was being replaced(17). In 1937 the government
deemed it necessary to introduce a subsidy of 50
per cent on lime bought by farmers. A steady improvement followed, but in 1943 50 per cent of

farmland in England and Wales was categorized as lime-deficient(18).

Table 1.3 summarizes one of the more reliable estimates of fertilizer consumption. In the case of all three plant foods the rate of increase in the 1940s is striking, and reflects deliberate Ministry of Agriculture influence in a decade when home food production was of the utmost importance, during the war and in the post-war period of acute economic difficulty.

In Table 1.4 some new estimates of farmers' expenditure on fertilizers are expressed as percentages of total costs of production. Both current and constant prices are used because over the whole period the price of fertilizers did not rise so rapidly as the prices of other factor inputs. As in Table 1.3, the rate of increase from 1935-37 to 1945-47 is apparent.

A broad survey of mechanization in arable farming suggests three main conclusions and the first is that much was gained in Britain from advances made overseas. Most of the improvements in tractor design came to this country from the United States as did the combined harvester and the automatic hay-baler. The best of new ditch-digging and drainage equipment was Scandinavian in origin, and one useful invention, a combined seed and fertilizer drill, originated in the Dominions. A second conclusion is that the triumph of the tractor should not be allowed to dominate the history of farm mechanization in Britain at this time. Most of the crucial developments in tractor design came between 1924 and 1939, yet only in the 1940s did it become the versatile form of draught power that we know today. In the thirties small tractors with pneumatic tyres were employed with success in root crop fields, in grassland improvement, and on hill farms, but such instances were notable examples rather than normal farm practice. The most advanced features of contemporary tractor design were not yet embodied in one single model, and the best of the new machines were more advanced than most of the standard models rolling off the production lines.

The mechanization of cereal harvesting involved much more than the displacement of horses by tractors. The combined harvester could only be used on a very limited scale in Britain until the threshing box was improved and efficient, smaller harvesters designed - these obstacles were not overcome until the 1940s. The mechanization of

Table 1.3: Estimated annual consumption of fertilizers for the United Kingdom expressed in terms of plant food (tons)

Year	Nitrogen (N)		Phosphate (P_2O_5)		Potash (K_2O)	
	(tons)	(%)	(tons)	(%)	(tons)	(%)
1903/14	n/a	–	191000	(=100)	n/a	–
1915/18	31400	(=100)	182000	(95)	n/a	–
1919/20	56800	(181)	232000	(121)	n/a	–
1921/31	42100	(134)	164000	(86)	43300	(=100)
1932/39	59400	(189)	172000	(90)	62500	(144)
1940/45	152500	(486)	283000	(148)	82000	(189)
1946/50	184600	(588)	390000	(204)	165700	(383)
1950	205000	(653)	430000	(225)	214600	(496)

Source: W. Gavin, 'The Way to Higher Crop Yields', Journal of the Ministry of Agriculture, LVIII No. 3 (June 1951) p. 106.

Table 1.4: Farmers' annual average expenditure on
fertilizers in England and Wales
expressed as percentage of expenditure on
total costs of production

Year	When measured in current prices (%)	When measured in constant 1911-13 prices (%)
1910-12	3.6	3.6
1915-17	4.9	4.1
1920-22	4.9	4.8
1925-27	3.4	4.8
1930-32	3.1	4.7
1935-37	3.5	5.4
1940-42	5.9	9.7
1945-47	6.8	14.7

Source: See Table 1.11 below.

hay-making owed a lot to tractor haulage but it
owed as much to the invention of the automatic
hay-baler, and to the discovery that the best quality hay is that which suffers the shortest necessary
interval between cutting and stacking. The biggest
problem in root crop harvesting remained unsolved
in spite of the advent of the tractor: how to design
a machine that would lift root crops from the ground
without damaging their tubers. Assuredly, the
story of farm mechanization from 1910 to 1950 contains more successes and problems than those encom-
passed by the coming of the tractor.
    The graph in Figure 1.2 portrays changes in
the agricultural horse population and the estimated tractor numbers. The increase in tractors
during both world wars is apparent. In 1914 there
were fewer than 600 at work, by 1918 the government
had imported and distributed over 10,000. During
the second war numbers increased from 52,000 in
1939 to 166,000 in 1945. On both occasions the
pace of mechanization was forced by means of the
close control assumed over farming practice by
the executive government,   at times when home

13

Figure 1.2

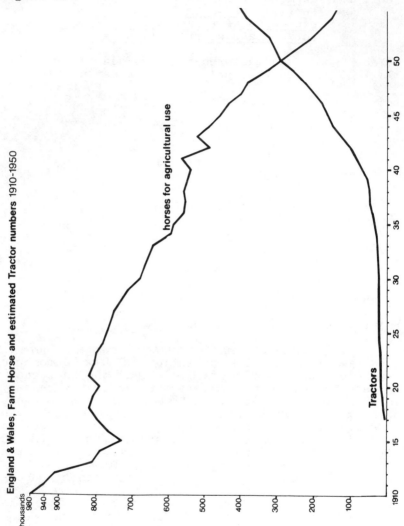

England & Wales, Farm Horse and estimated Tractor numbers 1910-1950

horses for agricultural use

Tractors

Sources: Ministry of Agriculture Fisheries and Food,
            A Century of Agricultural Statistics
            1866-1966 (1968), pp. 71, 129 and Farm
            Machinery Censuses for 1925, 1931 and 1935;
            Census of Production 1924, 1930 and 1935;
            Trade and Navigation Accounts, 1920-35;
            Jnl. Board of Agric. XXV (1918); Jnl. Min.
            Ag. XXVII (1920).

food production was of the utmost importance to an island at war.

Since a tractor can do more work than a horse in a given period of time it is necessary to consider the two forms of draught power in terms of available power, not merely in terms of numbers. An investigation by Britton and Keith(19) - summarized in Table 1.5 - led them to the conclusion that by 1934 the tractor had established its dominance over the horse as agriculture's main source of draught power. This view is an oversimplification because it ignores three necessary considerations. First, one must distinguish between potential horse-power and power actually utilized when doing farm work. Horses consistantly utilized a far higher proportion of their potential power than tractors during most field operations: a horse usually developed around 90 per cent of its available power, but the only time a tractor developed more than 63 per cent was when pulling a three-furrow plough(20). Thus in most farm tasks nothing like the full available power of the tractor's engine could be harnessed. A second consideration is the number of hours worked per year. The evidence for the 1930s(21) - scattered and fragmentary as it is - suggests that horses worked from 1500 to 1700 hours per year whereas tractors were used from 400 to 800 hours. Finally, it must be recognized that farmers used their tractors and horses as complementary rather than competing forms of draught power(22) until at least the early 'forties.

A tractor is an indivisible power unit which cannot be used in two places at once - unlike a team of horses. Thus the owner of a single tractor, reserving it for ploughing and heavy work, would be obliged to keep at least one or two horses for lighter tasks, haulage, and root crop harvesting (a process that involved both lifting the crop and hauling it from the field at lifting time). These considerations render inappropriate any notion that the tractor had supplanted the horse by 1934. In all probability this position was not reached until the mid-forties.

A third broad impression gained from a general survey of arable mechanization is that its great benefit was to speed up the pace of work at the busiest time of the year, when speed was essential to cope with the sheer volume of work and the threat of bad weather(23). Motorized harvesting and tractor ploughing enabled farmers to take advantage of brief spells of fine weather and press on

Table 1.5: Farm Draught Power Supplies (potential) in England and Wales 1908-48

Year	Tractors (000hp)	Horses (000hp)	Total Draught Power (000hp)
1908	-	964	964
1913	-	807	807
1925	340	773	1113
1931	364	667	1039
1937	810	555	1365
1939	950	549	1499
1942	1989	542	2531
1944	2982	485	3467
1946	3470	436	3906
1948	4372	384	4756

Source: The Farm Economist Vol. 6 no. 6 (1950), pp.163-71.

quickly with the late summer ingathering and early autumn ploughing; consequently, autumn sowing of cereals and beans became more widespread. Thus mechanization could be said to have given farmers a greater margin of defence against crop failure, since it is often possible to replace a damaged winter crop when there is usually no time to minister to a failed spring-sown one. The intensification of autumn tillage also conferred more power in the matter of weed control, for weeds establish themselves in arable fields in the interval between harvesting and the subsequent ploughing in preparation for next year's crop. By 1950 farmers were, of course, spending more on machinery than in 1910. Some new estimates are summarized in Table 1.6. The increase in expenditure on machinery (purchases and running costs) from 1935-37 to 1945-47 is striking, and is explained - again(24) - by the need to maximize home food production in the perilous circumstances of the 1940s.

Table 1.6: Farmers' expenditure on machinery in
England and Wales expressed as percentage
of total costs

Year (Annual Av)	When measured in current prices %	When measured in constant prices %
1910-12	7.3	7.5
1915-17	7.6	6.3
1920-22	9.9	8.0
1925-27	8.8	7.8
1930-32	7.3	6.7
1935-37	8.5	7.3
1940-42	15.0	13.7
1945-47	18.9	15.2

Sources: See Table 1.11 below.

Reference has been made(25) to the creation
of two Plant Breeding Institutes and a National
Institute of Agricultural Botany (NIAB) in 1919.
One important aspect of the NIAB's activities was
its work as the Ministry of Agriculture's official
seed-testing centre(26). Seeds were tested for
disease resistance, freedom from infection, and
varietal purity. The NIAB's recommendations formed
the basis of the Ministry's seed certification
scheme introduced in the 1920s. This work soon
became a routine branch of agricultural science,
but one of great practical importance to farmers
who now had access to better quality seed of a
guaranteed minimum standard.
In plant breeding three conspicuous successes
are worth recording. Varieties of cereals were
developed with shorter, thicker straw and, therefore, better standing qualities(27). New strains
of sugar beet were bred with a higher and more
stable sugar content(28). The Welsh Plant Breeding Station at Aberystwyth produced greatly improved
versions of most of the grasses necessary for a
good pasture, and their new varieties of wild white
clover were especially notable(29).
Crop disease is an ever-present problem.

Immunity to one strain of a disease can be bred
into a plant but, over the years, different strains
of that disease may develop in the fields. The
plant possessing resistance to one strain may well
remain susceptible to others: rust disease in cereals, especially wheat, is a case in point. By
1950 most of the common diseases of cereals and
root crops were still serious problems, but an
advance had been made with the reduction of wart
disease in potatoes(30), following the appearance
of new strains bred from South American stock,
and reflecting also the effects of the Ministry's
seed certification scheme. Dressing seeds with
a dust containing mercury salts afforded some de-
liverance from cereal diseases in the 1930s, and
later it was found to be effective against eel-
worm infestation in potatoes(31).

Most of the insecticides in use before 1939
were either simple chemical mixtures - lead arsen-
ate, copper sulphate, lime sulphur - or plant de-
rivatives based on derris root or pyrethrum. The
early 1940s marked the beginning of a new era in
plant protection, with the discovery and development of complex, synthetic chemicals possessed
of powerful insecticidal properties. The most
well-known (now notorious) example is DDT, introduced into this country from Switzerland in
1942(32). At about that time benzene hexochloride
was being developed independently in Britain -
at Jealott's Hill - and France(33). The discovery
of selective weed killers based on synthetic growth
regulators also emanated from Jealott's Hill in
the 1940s. Post-war publication of secret wartime trials led to the rapid acceptance of selective
hormone weed-killers. By 1952 over two million
acres of corn and grassland had been treated in
Britain alone(34).

Tangible though these advances in plant breeding and plant protection were, the problem of crop
health remained serious at mid-century. No easy
victories had been won.

The effects of scientific progress, including
mechanization, are indicated by the rise in recorded
crop yields summarized in Table 1.7. The increase
in root crop yields is more erratic than it is
for the cereals. Sugar beet is a special case
because it was fostered by government financial
assistance from 1924 to 1937(35). The low increase
in turnip and swede yields owes something to the
astonishingly heavy crops recorded in 1909 and
1910(36). Also, these two labour-intensive crops

Table 1.7: Yields per acre of main crops in England and Wales 1910-50

Annual Average	Wheat (cwt)	Barley (cwt)	Oats (cwt)	Potatoes (tons)	Turnips and Swedes (tons)	Sugar Beet (tons)
1909-11	17.7	16.1	14.3	6.5	13.4	–
1914-16	17.0	14.9	13.9	6.2	13.2	–
1919-21	17.1	14.3	12.8	5.6	11.1	6.8 (1921-23)
1924-26	17.4	15.6	15.2	6.0	13.2	8.2
1929-31	17.0	15.7	15.5	6.3	11.7	8.2
1934-36	18.1	16.6	15.7	6.5	10.3	9.7
1939-41	18.0	16.3	16.4	7.3	12.1	9.8
1944-46	19.1	18.1	16.7	6.9	13.3	9.2
1949-51	21.7	19.9	18.5	7.4	14.0	10.9
Increase 1909-11 to 1949-51 (in %)	22.6	23.6	29.4	13.8	4.5	60.3

Source: Ministry of Agriculture Fisheries and Food, A Century of Agricultural Statistics 1865-1966 (1968) pp 108-119.

declined in popularity in the 1920s when arable
farmers were squeezed by falling product prices
and rising labour costs(37), and they fell further
from favour later on when opinion turned against
the practice of including large quantities of roots
in standard animal rations(38).
Changes in acreage and production of the main
arable crops are summarized in Tables 1.8 and 1.9.
The main trends are an increase in area and output
from 1914-1916 to 1919-21, and again from the late
'thirties down to mid-century; and a contraction
in area and output from 1919-21 to the mid-'thirties. These fluctuations reflect four major influences which must now be identified.
During both world wars the need to reduce
food imports impelled an expansion of arable farming. In the difficult years following 1945 Britain suffered an acute shortage of foreign exchange,
and the need to economize on food imports remained
scarcely less urgent than in war-time. Hence,
by 1949-51 main crop acreage was larger than in
1909-11. Apart from the influence of war (and
post-war dislocation), government policy began
to revive arable farming in the mid-thirties. The
Wheat Act of 1932 provided a subsidy on home-grown
wheat in order to re-expand the acreage to its
pre-1914 level. This was achieved, but largely
at the expense of barley and oats, so a subsidy
for producers of barley and oats was included in
the Agriculture Act of 1937(39).
The contraction of arable acreage and output
from 1919-21 to the mid-thirties is mainly explained
by the world surplus of farm produce - particularly
grain - existing at that time. In consequence
agricultural prices were low, but until 1932 Britain
remained, largely, a free-trade country and her
farmers were vulnerable to cheap grain imports.
The return to protection in 1932 did not entirely
solve the problem for it was protection with Imperial preference, which left British farmers open
to competition from cheap Commonwealth food(40).
Another factor working against arable farming in
the inter-war period was a discernible change in
the nation's diet. In spite of heavy unemployment,
average real per capita income was rising between
1925 and 1938(41). This increase induced or supported a change in dietary habits: consumption
of the basic energy-supplying foods like bread
and potatoes declined, whilst consumption of fruit,
vegetables, livestock and dairy produce advanc-
ed(42).

The main trends in arable output and acreage have been identified and explained. An indication of how these trends affected the relative importance of arable production in total agricultural output is given in Table 1.10.

Four main conclusions may be drawn from this brief, broad survey of science and practice in English arable farming. First, in most areas of agricultural science progress in this country was aided by research and developments overseas. This was not a one-way trade; in soil science, fertilizer studies, and grassland research Britain was a world leader, and important advances in plant breeding, plant protection, and farm machinery were conceived and completed in this country.

A second conclusion is that the effects of war were decidedly mixed. The finance of research was adversely affected, and the conduct of it disrupted, in 1914-18 and 1939-45. However, during both wars existing arrangements for research were scrutinized with a new urgency, weaknesses were identified and remedial action taken. The effects of the first war in this respect have been discussed above(43); during the second war, when two government reports criticized the arrangements for research and advisory work in agricultural engineering(44), improvements were swiftly made(45). Furthermore, both wars had an improving influence upon standards of arable farming. The use of machinery and modern fertilizers became more widespread, and farmers became more concerned with issues of crop improvement and crop protection. This was due to the close control over farming practice assumed by the Ministry of Agriculture and exercised through the County War Agricultural Executive Committees (CWAECs)(46). The CWAECs worked mainly by persuasion and advice but, in extreme cases, persistently unco-operative owners or occupiers could be dispossessed.

A third salient point is that the Ministry of Agriculture played a major part in bringing the results of scientific research onto the farm in peacetime, too. Reference has been made above(47) to subsidies and other schemes for the encouragement of good husbandry. In addition, the Ministry's multifarious advisory and information leaflets, and its monthly Journal, were important sources for communicating to the farmer details of modern, best-practice methods. The volume and variety of the Ministry's own advisory work must not be forgotten when one encounters the standard crit-

Table 1.8: Acreage of main crops and temporary
pasture in England and Wales 1910-50
(000 acres)

Annual Average	Wheat	Barley	Oats	A Total Cereals	Potatoes
1909-11	1791	1475	2049	5313 (56)	422
1914-16	1963	1356	2034	5353 (58)	451
1919-21	2024	1528	2328	5880 (60)	526
1924-26	1546	1260	1923	4829 (55)	481
1929-31	1291	1056	1762	4109 (51)	464
1934-36	1745	824	1414	3983 (53)	469
1939-41	1840	1157	1961	4958 (60)	589
1944-46	2409	1903	998	5310 (50)	991
1949-51	2119	1747	1808	5674 (52)	842

Percentage
change

1909-11 to 1949-51	+18.3	+18.4	-11.8	+6.8	+99.5

Source: Agricultural Statistics 1866-1966,
pp. 97-103

Table 1.8 (contd.)

Turnip & Swedes	Sugar Beet	B Total Root Crops	C Temporary Pasture	D Total
1121	–	1543 (16)	2702 (28)	9560 (100)
972	–	1423 (15)	2498 (27)	9274 (100)
956	4	1486 (15)	2462 (25)	9828 (100)
802	68	1351 (16)	2596 (30)	8676 (100)
664	270	1398 (17)	2498 (31)	8005 (100)
489	371	1329 (18)	2205 (29)	7517 (100)
443	335	1367 (16)	1969 (24)	8294 (100)
464	416	1871 (18)	3383 (32)	10564 (100)
322	416	1580 (14)	3690 (34)	10944 (100)
-71.2	+10300	+2.4	+36.6	+14.5

Table 1.9: Production of main crops in England and Wales 1910-50 (000 tons)

Annual Average	Wheat	Barley	Oats	Potatoes	Turnips & Swedes	Sugar Beet
1909-11	1588	1185	1464	2748	15060	–
1914-16	1671	1013	1415	2772	12748	–
1919-21	1726	1095	1489	2947	10653	75
1924-26	1342	980	1456	2891	10573	567
1929-31	1101	836	1367	2928	7737	2237
1934-36	1583	682	1111	3044	4942	3588
1939-41	1650	931	1599	4294	5363	3252
1944-46	2308	1720	1859	6819	6197	3802
1949-51	2293	1743	1667	6199	4476	4474
Percentage Change 1909-11 to 1949-51	+44.4	+47.1	+13.9	+125.6	-70.3	+5865.3

Source: Agricultural Statistics 1866-1966, pp. 108-119.

Table 1.10: Value of Farm Crops as a percentage of
value of Gross Agricultural Output

England and Wales		United Kingdom	
1910	31.5	1939-40	18.3
1924-5	24.1	1940-41	22.3
1925-6	20.6	1941-42	27.3
1926-7	22.5	1942-43	31.1
1927-8	21.6	1943-44	30.7
1928-9	19.5	1944-45	26.8
1929-30	17.4	1945-46	27.4
1930-31	18.5	1946-47	24.1
1931-32	18.1	1947-48	20.0
1932-33	14.9	1948-49	22.8
1933-34	15.6	1949-50	19.3
1934-35	17.8	1950-51	21.0
1935-36	17.3		
1936-37	18.0		
1937-38	15.7		
1938-39	14.5		

Source: Agricultural Statistics 1910-55.

icisms levelled at the under-financed and under-
staffed county and provincial advisory services
in the inter-war period(48).

Finally, no-one will be surprised to learn
that in 1950 farmers were using more fertilizers,
more machinery, and less labour than their pre-
decessors of 1910. However, the price of these
three items did not increase at the same rate over
the whole period. A new estimate is summarized
in Table 1.11:(49) fertilizer prices rose less,
and wages rose more, than other costs of production.
Accordingly, when expenditure is estimated in current prices, the increased expenditure on fertilizers understates the increase in fertilizer usage,
and the increased expenditure on labour does not
reflect the substantial decline which actually
took place in the farm labour force(50). This point
should not be laboured, but many of the published
statistics usually refer to current prices only(51).

From 1910 to 1950 arable farmers lived through
two world wars, a severe depression in the inter-
war period, and a phase of acute economic difficulty
in the late 1940s. When one reflects upon those
times, then the improvement in farming methods,
and the expansion of crop production, appear as
considerable achievements(52).

Table 1.11: Farmers' expenditure on selected inputs in England and Wales 1910-1950

Annual Average	Fertilizer		Machinery		Labour (a)		Total Expenditure*
	(£mn)	(%)	(£mn)	(%)	(£mn)	(%)	(£mn)
Current Prices							
1910-12	4.5	(3.6)	9.2	(7.3)	44.5	(35.3)	126.0
1915-17	7.8	(4.9)	12.0	(7.6)	53.5	(33.8)	158.2
1920-22	11.9	(4.9)	24.2	(9.9)	100.6	(41.3)	243.4
1925-27	7.2	(3.4)	18.3	(8.8)	76.6	(36.6)	209.1
1930-32	5.8	(3.1)	13.7	(7.3)	73.3	(39.3)	186.4
1934-37	6.7	(3.5)	16.5	(8.5)	70.5	(36.5)	193.3
1940-42	14.7	(5.9)	37.3	(15.0)	105.1	(42.3)	248.6
1945-47	23.7	(6.8)	65.3	(18.9)	163.9	(47.3)	346.2
Constant Prices (1911-13)							
1910-12	4.6	(3.6)	9.6	(7.5)	45.5	(35.4)	128.7
1915-17	5.0	(4.1)	7.7	(6.3)	40.9	(33.6)	121.6
1920-22	5.7	(4.8)	9.5	(8.0)	40.1	(33.8)	118.6
1925-27	6.4	(4.8)	10.4	(7.8)	38.6	(29.1)	132.8
1930-32	6.1	(4.7)	8.7	(6.7)	36.0	(28.3)	129.9
1934-37	7.5	(5.4)	10.1	(7.3)	34.4	(24.9)	138.0
1940-42	11.6	(9.7)	16.4	(13.7)	32.9	(27.4)	120.1
1945-47	18.2	(14.7)	18.8	(15.2)	34.2	(27.7)	123.6

Sources: Agricultural Statistics 1910-50; E. Ojala, Agriculture and Economic Progress Oxford (1952)

(a) includes a wage input to farmers.
* animal feed, store animals, seeds, rent, plus the three listed here.

NOTES

1. In the period under discussion figures of
    average yield per acre for the main crops,
    based on estimates sent in by official 'crop
    reporters' throughout the country, were often
    regarded as being too low. Certainly they
    were consistently below a series produced
    each year by The Times, using a similar, but
    more extensive, network of crop reporters.
    The early censuses of agricultural production
    in the 1920s have an aura of uncertainty about
    them too, because the returns from which they
    were derived were furnished on a voluntary
    basis, thus the farmers making returns con-
    stituted a biased sample of the whole. Three
    serious omissions are the lack of any infor-
    mation about the quality and quantity of grass
    grazed by livestock throughout the growing
    season, the absence of estimates of the agri-
    cultural wages bill for the years before 1936,
    and the paucity of farm machinery censuses
    before 1942. These few examples make it clear
    that one should constantly bear in mind the
    deficiencies of the agricultural statistics.
    D.K. Britton and K.E. Hunt 'Agriculture' in
    M.G. Kendall (ed.), The Sources and Nature
    of the Statistics of the United Kingdom Vol.1
    (1952) pp. 35-74 contains a full discussion
    of the deficiencies of British agricultural
    statistics.
2. Board of Agriculture and Fisheries, Report
    on the Distribution of Grants for Agricultural
    Education and Research 1910/11, Cd 6025 (1911)
    p.xiii.
3. Development Commission, Tenth Report of the
    Development Commissioners for the Year ended
    31st March 1920; with a Review of the Work
    of the Commission during the Past Ten Years,
    (1920) p. 1.
4. Development Commission, Fourteenth Report
    of the Development Commissioners for the Year
    ended 31st March, 1924, (1924) p. 2.
5. Development Commission, Tenth Report, (1920)
    pp. 21, 37, 38. Ministry of Reconstruction,
    Report of the Agricultural Policy Sub-Com-
    mittee of the Reconstruction Committee, Cd
    9079 (1918) para. 166, p. 49. Development
    Commission, Fifteenth Report, (1925) p. 95.
    T.H. Middleton, Food Production in War,
    (Oxford 1923) p. 226.

6. Parliamentary Papers (a) Civil Appropriation Accounts 1911/12 - 1950/51; (b) Development Fund Accounts 1912/13 - 1924/25; (c) Accounts of the Agricultural Research Council 1931/32 - 1942/3; (d) Annual Reports of the Development Commissioners 1910/11 - 1938/9.

7. From the Sources cited in note 6 above it is possible to divide expenditure on the state research network into capital grants and current grants. Capital grants have been deflated by a price index of non-residential buildings and works, re-based to 1911-13 = 100, see C.H. Feinstein, Statistical Tables of National Income, Expenditure and Output of the United Kingdom 1855-1965, (Cambridge, 1976), T137. Current grants have been deflated by a composite index of administrative and executive grade civil service salaries, re-based to 1911-13 = 100, see G. Routh, 'Civil Service Pay, 1875 to 1950', Economica N.S. XXI (1954) p. 216.

8. For a full account of these early developments see V.E. Parke, Billingham - The First Ten Years, (1957).

9. ICI Ltd., Enterprise and Responsibility; ICI in Agriculture, (1959) pp. 8-10.

10. See below page 10.

11. ICI Ltd., Jealott's Hill, the Agricultural Research Station of Imperial Chemical Industries Limited; a Record of Twenty-Five Years (1953) contains a short history and conveys an impression of the range and quality of agricultural research at Jealott's Hill from 1928 to 1953 (in this connection see also note 12 below).

12. E.J. Russell, A History of Agricultural Science in Great Britain, 1620-1954 (1966) pp. 325-31. This excellent book also indicates the high regard in which Jealott's Hill was held by agricultural scientists - see pp. 440-3, 462-4.

13. See the annual review published in the Journal of the Royal Agricultural Society of England from 1931 to 1950 (and after): 'The Farmer's Guide to Agricultural Research'.

14. A.W. Menzies Kitchin, 'Local Administration of Agricultural Policy' in D.N. Chester (ed.) Lessons of the British War Economy (Cambridge, 1952), pp. 241-2.

15. H.T. Williams, Principles for British Agricultural Policy (Oxford, 1960), p. 31.

16. J. Porter, 'Liming in Herefordshire', Journal of the Ministry of Agriculture XXVII (1920/21), p. 157. B.H. Bedell, 'The Need for Lime and How to Meet it', Jnl. Min. Ag. XXVIII (1921/2), p. 200. D. Turner, 'Lime Survey in the West Midland Counties', Jnl.Min.Ag. XXXIII (1926/7), pp. 316-7.

17. B.H. Bedell, Jnl. Min. Ag. XXXVIII (1921/22), p. 200.

18. G.W. Robinson, 'The Use of Lime', Jnl. Royal Ag. Soc. 104 (1943), p. 139.

19. D.K. Britton and I.F. Keith, 'A Note on the Statistics of Farm Power Supplies in Great Britain', The Farm Economist VI. 6 (1950), pp. 163-70.

20. R.A. Dudman, 'Of Horses and Tractors', The Farm Economist V. 7 (1950), pp. 181-8 especially 182.

21. A.J. Marval, 'Tractor Working Costs, 1930-35' The Farm Economist II. 8 (1937), p. 158; J. Wyllie, Investigation into Farming Costs of Production and Financial Results XXXVIII; The Cost of Horse Labour and Tractor Work - 1936/7 to 1944/5. (Wye College, Department of Economics, 1946); J.R. Lee, Studies in Power Farming II: The Cost of Tractor Work, (The Agricultural Economics Research Institute, Oxford, 1936).

22. S.J. Wright, 'Mechanical Row Crop Cultivation', Jnl. Min. Ag., XLV (1938/9), pp. 103-7.

23. The Times, August 30, 1915, p. 4, 'Machinery on the Land'; Ministry of Agriculture and Fisheries, Report of the Departmental Committee on Agricultural Machinery, Cmd. 506 (1920) p. 6; The Times, Sept. 22, 1919 p.5, 'Farm Machinery'; A.W. Oldershaw, 'Stubble Cleaning', Jnl. Min. Ag. XXXVII (1930/1) pp. 423-5.

24. See above, pages 11 and 16.

25. See above page 1.

26. Russell, Agricultural Science, pp. 345-6; The Times, April 13, 1931 p. 18 'Seed Potatoes'; The Times, August 17, 1931 p. 15 'Better Seeds'; F. Carnshaw, A Description of the Recommended Varieties of Wheat and Barley, (National Institute of Agricultural Botany, Cambridge, 1948).

27. G.D.H. Bell, 'Some British Plant-Breeding Problems', Agricultural Progress XXV (1950), pp. 1-10.

28. D.H. Robinson, 'Tillage Crops', in J.A. Hanley

(ed.) Progressive Farming I (1949), pp. 128-9.
29. Bell, Agricultural Progress XXV, pp. 1-10;
Political and Economic Planning. Report on
Agricultural Research in Great Britain (1938),
p. 82.
30. G.D. Bell, 'Crops and Plant Breeding', The
Farmer's Guide to Agricultural Research in
1937. J.R. Ag.S.E. 99 (1938), p. 129.
31. W.C. Moore, 'Modern Developments in Crop Protection', J.R. Ag. S.E. 116 (1955), p. 20.
32. For an interesting account of the discovery
and early development of Diphenyl - Dich-
loro - Trichlorethane see T.F. West and G.A.
Campbell, DDT; the Synthetic Insecticide
(1946).
33. ICI Ltd., Research in Agriculture; a Record
of Twenty-six Years (1954), p. 23.
34. Ibid. pp. 25/6.
35. For an account, see Viscount Astor and B.
Seebohm Rowntree, British Agriculture; the
Principles of Future Policy (1938), pp. 90-106.
36. The yields were 15.7 tons per acre in 1909
and 15.6 in 1910. These were the highest
annual figures returned in the entire period
from 1884 to 1950, and were not exceeded until
the decade of the fifties. See Ministry of
Agriculture Fisheries and Food, Department
of Agriculture and Fisheries for Scotland,
A Century of Agricultural Statistics: Great
Britain 1866-1966 (1968), Table 61 pp. 118-19.
37. Ibid. Table 38 p. 85, Table 27 p. 65.
38. V.H. Beynon, 'Some Considerations on the Feeding of Dairy Cows', Jnl. Min. Ag. 59 (1952/3),
p. 302.
39. These matters are discussed in E.H. Whetham,
The Agrarian History of England and Wales,
Volume VIII: 1914-39 (Cambridge, 1979),
pp. 243-4, 255, 258-9, 260-2, 284, 313, 327.
40. Williams, Agricultural Policy, pp. 11-20.
41. Feinstein, National Income, T42.
42. Williams, Agricultural Policy, p. 20.
43. See pages 5-6 and 9 above.
44. First Report of the Agricultural Improvement
Council for England and Wales (1944), pp.9-10;
Report of the Committee on Post-War Agricultural Education in England and Wales, Cmd.
6433 (1943), pp. 26-7.
45. The National Institute for Research in Agricultural Engineering was reformed, improved,
and transferred from Oxford to Yorkshire,
in 1942. When the National Agricultural

Advisory Service was created in 1946, advisory officers in farm machinery were appointed - there had been no such posts in the Provincial Advisory Service before 1939.

46. For an account of the work of the CWAECs see Whetham, Agrarian History, pp. 91-4, 97-108 (for 1914-18); Menzies Kitchin, in Chester (ed.) British War Economy, pp. 239-49 (for 1939-45).

47. See pages 9-10 and 17-18.

48. See, for instance, PEP, Agricultural Research, pp. 55-70.

49. 'Total expenditure' comprises fertilizers, machinery, labour (including an imputed wage to farmers), purchased animal feeds, store animals, seeds, and rent. Each item has been deflated by an appropriate price index.

50. For the details see Agricultural Statistics 1866-1966, Table 26. p. 62.

51. For example, Agricultural Statistics 1866-1966, Table 32 pp. 76-7, Table 33 p. 78; Agricultural Statistics 1925-50.

52. In the summer of 1980 earlier versions of this paper were given at the Modern History Group's Seminar, University of Surrey, and the Nutritionists' and Historians' Seminar, Queen Elizabeth College, University of London. I am grateful to members of both groups for their most helpful criticisms and informed comments. I must thank Gareth Hughes, of Kingston Polytechnic, and John Robertson, of the Milk Marketing Board, for expert advice on quantitative methods.

2. THE IMPACT OF MODERN FOOD TECHNOLOGY ON NUTRITION IN 20TH CENTURY BRITAIN

MAGNUS PYKE

After half a century of belief in the potency of science to influence social affairs, now is a good moment to ask, when the initial euphoria stimulated by early discoveries is passing, whether science has studied the nutritional needs of different types of individuals for health and whether scientific understanding has been applied to develop technological processes of food production by which people's nutritional needs can be met. It would be foolish to suggest that modern food technology has had no impact at all on the nutritional status in Britain, nevertheless its influence has been less significant and less direct than was at one time assumed.

The state of nutrition, whether in twentieth-century Britain or anywhere else, is influenced by a number of factors, of which the level of nutritional knowledge and technological expertise of food manufacturers are only two and, though important, not the most important. We must, for example, rank above them, firstly, the level of prosperity in the community as a whole, the social structure, particularly so far as it affects the relative economic levels of the rich and the poor, the efficiency of the system for the transport and distribution of food and, perhaps most important of all, the standards of hygiene both within the community as maintained by food producers, processors and distributors. Yet even though it is possible to conceive a society, particularly one possessing a good knowledge of nutritional science, enjoying a high standard of nutritional well-being without the benefit of modern food technology at all, food technology can undoubtedly be seen to have made a contribution to the nutritional status of the nation, if only as part of economic activity and irrespective of what aspects of food processing are specifically directed towards nutritional ends.

Nutritional status early in the twentieth century

Whatever impact modern food technology has exerted on nutrition could be assessed in three ways. Firstly, we could consider what was wrong with the nutritional status of the population early in the century before today's technological processes came into existence and try to assess to what extent they had been instrumental in ameliorating the situation. Alternatively, it might be possible to reach some conclusion as to whether the state of nutrition now, under the circumstances of modern life and an increased population, could only have become possible because of the successes of the technological processes developed in the food industry. A third approach would be to look for evidence of harm which could legitimately be attached to food processing affecting the nutrition of people now but not seen before modern methods were introduced.

Early in the century, although there was indeed scope for nutritional improvement, there is little evidence to suggest that malnutrition attributable to the inadequacies of food technology was a major public-health problem. The upper classes who sent their sons to the prestigious private schools, which the English so perversely describe as 'public', were taller and heavier for their age than the children of working-class parents, as shown by, among others, the Glasgow education authorities who have collected records of heights and weights systematically since 1914. The steady increase in the measurements and the corresponding narrowing of the gap between rich and poor children, taken as a measure of improved nutrition among the latter, must, however, be attributed more directly to the parallel growth in the influence of the Socialist Party and the corresponding change in the economic status of the working people enabling them to buy more food and their children to obtain school dinners, among other social benefits, rather than to any particular technological innovation by food manufacturers. It is true that Moynahan has pointed out that the acceleration of the onset of puberty as well as the increase in stature in all classes in the industrial nations began in 1870(1), precisely the time when roller-milling of flour was introduced. Since then there has been a progressive decrease in the fibre content of the diet concomitant with the improvement in stature and earlier puberty. Cellulose is a major component of fibre in cereals. It is, therefore, surprising that so little attention has been paid to its binding capacity for trace minerals, especially since this property has been exploited with considerable success in the analytical process of paper chromatography. Part of the explanation may lie in the fact that current understanding of the role of zinc deficiency in the diet retarding growth and delaying puberty in children had to await technical developments of a satisfactory assay of the metal. There is now increasing evidence (Reinhold et al) to suggest that increased availability of zinc may have played a major role in the striking improvement in growth and physique accompanying the introduction of bread made from the white flour which became available to the British community following the introduction of the new technology of milling(2). It would be bizarre if this turned out to be so in view, not only of the attention now being given to what are thought to be the beneficial properties of fibre, if not as a source of nutrients at least as a pharmaceutical agent, but also to the concentration of interest on the relative vitamin content of roller-milled flour in comparison with the product of the pre-nineteenth century technology of flour milling.

The dramatic nutritional discoveries early in the twentieth century, particularly of the existence of vitamins, made a deep impression on the scientific community and the general public alike. Now that a half-century has elapsed, it can be seen that both groups - the scientists and the public - formed an incorrect opinion about the relevance of many of these discoveries to the nutritional well-being of the community. For example, the attention paid to the ascorbic acid analysis of fruit and vegetables, the educational effort expended towards the cooking of cabbage, and the supplementation of a variety of manufactured foods and drinks with vitamins of all sorts was not reflected in any measurable evidence of demonstrable improvement in public health attributable thereto. This is hardly surprising in a community where scurvy due to lack of ascorbic acid over a prolonged space of time had ceased to be a problem since the introduction of turnips into agriculture in the eighteenth century, quite apart from the

general consumption of potatoes more than a century
earlier. Similar ambiguity surrounds the attention
paid to other vitamins. The concern felt about
the vitamin B content of bread is a good example
of this. Prior to the development of modern food
technology, white bread was prized as a luxury
which the rich only were able to enjoy. The development of modern milling techniques which took
place mainly, as has already been noted, in the
nineteenth century but reached its present level
of flexibility and control only within the last
sixty years, made white bread readily available
to the entire community, rich and poor alike. Although, due to the quirks of fashion, a minority,
mainly of the middle and upper classes, have developed a taste for bread made from more coarsely
ground flour, a large majority of British consumers
show a firmly held preference for white bread.
This preference has been maintained in the face
of urgent propaganda by those who feel concern
for the public welfare and favour the higher concentration of thiamine, riboflavin, niacin, pyridoxin
and other vitamins in brown bread. Indeed, in
the light of the fact that synthetic thiamine is
readily available at a comparatively low price,
this vitamin is by law added to white flour used
for bread making.

Yet in a review of the impact of modern food
technology on the nutritional state of the British
public, it is difficult to find evidence to support
the conclusion that before the twentieth century
there were specific signs of a deficiency of any
of the B vitamins. In countries where the diet
is significantly lacking in thiamine, the disease
beri beri occurs. Beri beri is never seen in Great
Britain, except as a medical curiosity as a result
of advanced alcoholism where the patient has virtually given up eating food. Nor have significant
indications of deficiencies of other B vitamins
been identified either before or during the twentieth century. It is difficult to evade the conclusion that the unsatisfactory physique of recruits
enrolled to fight the Boer War in 1901 was more
directly due to poverty with all its associated
circumstances of bad housing and insufficient food
rather than to a shortage of one vitamin or another.
It can also be argued that the continuation of
the same progression of events was demonstrated
in the facts that came to light when the physique
of men entering the armed services again became

a public issue in 1914, at the start of World War
I and again in 1939 at the outbreak of World War
II. On each occasion, as in 1901, while there
was some evidence to imply that some of the men
belonging to the poorer classes - what we are
accustomed today to describe as 'under-privileged'
- appeared to be undernourished, little solid evidence is available to imply that specific nutritional deficiencies existed which could have been directly benefited or harmed by developments in modern food technology.

But even if it is difficult to particularize
as to whether one specific nutrient or the lack
of it in a selected product of modern food technology influenced the nutritional well-being of
the British public as the twentieth century progressed, it is clear that the influence of technological developments in food processing will
undoubtedly have influenced the composition of
the diet as a whole, the availability of the separate articles of the diet and, perhaps most important of all, the cost of food. Thomson has
recently pointed out that up till 1928, when Professor E.P. Cathcart the distinguished professor
of physiology at Glasgow University published his
popular book on nutrition, the connection between
income and nutrition had not been accepted as applying under the economic circumstances of the
times(3). Cathcart wrote, 'It has been our experience, as the result of repeated dietary studies,
that one of the most prominent contributory factors
towards defective and deficient dietaries is not
so much the inadequacy of the income as its faulty
expenditure'(4).

Eight years later, in 1936, John Boyd Orr
published his book, Food, Health and Income(5).
In this he gave evidence to show that the diet
eaten by casual workers and their families was
less satisfactory and contained less fruit, vegetables, dairy products and meat than did the diet
of semi-skilled workers, who themselves ate a less
plentiful and varied diet than did the families
of skilled workers. Although Orr's work was restricted to a study of what people ate, he suggested
that other evidence available at the time together
with calculations of the nutritional content of
the diets surveyed implied that ten per cent of
the working population had insufficient money to
enable them to buy a diet nutritionally adequate
to supply their needs for full health.

After the lapse of more than forty years,

it is difficult to judge whether there was at that time sufficient evidence to justify this conclusion. A number of extensive surveys were carried out following the publication of Orr's report to examine the effect of supplementing the diet of schoolchildren in various parts of the country with milk distributed to the schools. Although the groups receiving milk grew somewhat more than those serving as controls, the difference between them was narrow and it is not easy to judge the statistical validity of the experimental results. Thomson has pointed out that at the time the trials were initiated there was a surplus of milk for which the Ministry of Agriculture was anxious to find a means of disposal.

Milk technology and health

Milk is undoubtedly a nourishing food and is particularly important in the feeding of infants and young children even though there remains some area of ambiguity about its true significance for schoolchildren under the conditions of twentieth-century Britain. In my view, one of the most important technological innovations of the century in the area of food affecting the health of children was the general introduction of pasteurization. Although this drastically reduced the number of cases of tuberculosis of the joints in children and reduced the incidence of other infectious diseases in the community, its influence on nutrition as such can only be claimed to be indirect and rendering milk safe to feed infants and young children, for whom there is good evidence that milk, distributed either liquid or as a dry powder, possesses nutritional significance. It is, therefore, interesting to note that throughout the 1930s and 1940s a violent campaign was waged by people opposed to pasteurization to prevent its introduction. Looking back, a historian could feel justified in deducing that the basis of this perverse campaign was, in the main, a misunderstanding of the then newly discovered facts of nutritional science and of their relevance to public health, those opposed to the pasteurization of milk often basing their arguments on its allegedly destructive effect on some of its minor nutrients. No serious effort was ever made to identify the ills this damage was deemed to have produced or show how their avoidance counterbalanced the demonstrably beneficial effect of pasteurization. I have described this campaign in some detail elsewhere(6).

If pasteurization can reasonably be judged to be one area of milk technology affecting, even if indirectly, the nutrition of the community, a further technological process of nutritional significance has been dehydration. The first technique to be adopted was roller drying. In this process, a thin film of milk is continuously applied to a steam-heated roller. As the roller revolves, the dried film is removed by means of a scraper. Considerable study was required before the appropriate temperature and time in contact with the roller were so adjusted as to produce powder capable of ready and approximately complete reconstitution to yield for use a liquid of acceptable flavour. An alternative process of spray drying was to cause fine globules of milk to fall through a current of warm air blown upwards from the bottom of a tall conical vessel. By the time the liquid droplets of milk reached the base of the vessel they had become a fine dry powder.

During the first two or three decades of the century, milk powder, whether produced by roller-drying or spray-drying, constituted the main ingredient of the artificial baby foods which quite rapidly increased in popularity. Rickets, which at that time constituted a considerable public health hazard and to which bottle-fed babies had been especially prone, was quickly overcome by the discovery in 1924 that vitamin D, now called cholecalciferol, could be produced by the irradiation of ergosterol.

Probably of all the influences of modern food technology on the British community this was the most important and dramatic. It is perhaps worth recalling that, important though it was, it was restricted to the diet of infants and children, a minority so far as food supplies are concerned. Yet by knowledge becoming available to improve the nutrition of this sensitive group, the incidence of bent and crippled adults, once so saddening a phenomenon in the crowded working-class districts of northern Britain, was drastically reduced together with that of malformed women for whom childbearing had once been dangerous both to themselves and to the children they found it so difficult to bear. Prior to 1900, in many of the great industrial cities, not only of Great Britain but of the world as a whole, be it in Glasgow, Vienna or Lahore, up to seventy-five per cent of the children of the poorer classes were affected(7). By

the end of World War II, when not only were the
dried milk preparations produced by food technologists for commercial firms and for the Government
alike, reinforced with cholecalciferol, but so
also were numerous cereal preparations, rusks,
breakfast foods and the like. Rickets, from having
been a matter of serious concern at the beginning
of the century, had within fifty years dwindled
to the status of a rarity which many paediatricians
seldom or never saw. It is true that in 1952,
Lightwood described a new disease of infants, idio-
pathic hypercalcaemia. Between 1953 and 1955,
two hundred and sixty cases were observed in various
centres. Some of these were serious and a few
fatal. Nevertheless by 1957, when the amount of
cholecalciferol incorporated in infant-feeding
mixtures and the like was reduced, the very significant benefits of this development in food technology, namely the incorporation of chemical compounds with vitamin activity, were being obtained
to the clear advantage of the community.

But the direct effect of modern food technology, derived from the advances in the techniques
of milk dehydration, progress in the understanding
of the nutritional needs of infants and the provision of such needs by the supplementation of powdered milk with synthetic nutrients, is only one
aspect of the impact of this area of food manufacture on the welfare of the British community. I
have already touched on the truism that poverty
is, as it has been throughout history, a major
influence on nutritional status. But poverty itself is a concept which is more difficult to define
than is generally imagined in the complex industrial
society existing in modern Britain. A general
definition of poverty is the condition of possessing a money income insufficient to provide
the standard of living individuals consider they
need in the sort of society in which they live.
In the twentieth-century Britain we are considering,
people can suffer from genuine poverty by which
their nutritional well-being is affected while
possessing colour-television sets and three-piece
suites of furniture for which weekly payments must
be made. It is to protect themselves against such
poverty that in a substantial proportion of the
families in industrial communities both husband
and wife go out to work five days out of seven
to earn the money by which their families' nutritional status is to be maintained. The food processors, through whose efforts enriched dehydrated-

milk mixtures are today available, make it possible for women who would otherwise need to stay at home breast-feeding their babies so to support the economic status of their families by working.

It has been estimated that about eighty-five per cent of all the infants in Great Britain, and in the United States as well, receive no significant amount of human milk and that these many millions of babies have been reared successfully on mixtures based on cows' milk, the majority of which are the product of modern food technology(9). A significant part of the success of bottle feeding is due to the technological and educational status of the British community where clean water is universally available, women possess the facilities allowing them to prepare their baby's feeds, and the education enabling them to understand the instructions telling them how to do so. At the same time, the freedom which allows mothers to contribute to the economic status of the families of which they are members - or, by definition, allows them to choose otherwise - protects them from the inadequate nutrition which is so commonly associated with poverty.

Apprehensions of nutritional damage

The progress of the twentieth century has been marked by a steady and, in the main, continuous rise in the standard of living of the community as marked by the increase in the general availability of the products of technology by which life is made more comfortable, varied and rich. It is not only television sets that have penetrated to all classes of society. The ownership of motor cars, refrigerators, telephones, vacuum cleaners and electric razors; foreign travel made possible by cheap air fares; and improvement in the conditions of work - all these have become possible because of advances in technology. The cost of making all this available to the ordinary citizen depends on a parallel increase in the economic productivity of each. It is this necessity for economic effectiveness that is one of the factors leading to the disappearance of shops with one assistant serving just one customer, and their replacement by supermarkets. To meet the demands of this method of distribution, packaged 'convenience' foods needed to be developed. Similarly, for low-cost catering, there were developed so-called 'fast' foods.

Quite early in the nineteenth century, when the industrial revolution was in progress and Great Britain was changing from the mainly rural society of the eighteenth century into an urban one, attention was directed to the purity and wholesomeness of the food offered for sale. This has continued. But whereas in the nineteenth century and early in the twentieth it was a matter of gross adulteration, for example, alum mixed with flour or, as the music-hall song put it, 'Little drops of water, little grains of sand/ Make the milkman merry and the grocer grand.' in more recent times, when such adulteration was a thing of the past, regulations were promulgated insisting on the declaration of the presence of such approved and tested ingredients as had been incorporated.

Not recognising the names or knowing the origins of the various substances - those added to keep the packed food moist, to enhance its flavour or colour, to maintain a desired consistency or to prevent oil and water from separating out - the consumers who, through their own delegates, had required the components to be listed, began to feel unease. It became popular wisdom to believe that the products of food technology were in some way unwholesome. Though their precise harmfulness or their alleged lack of nutrients is not specified, there grew a popular belief in their responsibility for the 'diseases of civilization'. What these diseases are is not always particularized. Obesity is often mentioned. Since the basic cause of obesity is the consumption of more food than the daily activities of the consumer demand, modern food technology, by which many of the foods on the market are produced and distributed, can be blamed, although who would prefer a situation in which food was scarce? Similarly, diabetes, although associated with a high level of nutrition and itself being a breakdown in carbohydrate metabolism, can more appropriately be associated with an unwise selection of food and, perhaps, too much rather than with the nature and composition of a particular article. Coronary heart disease too, is associated with obesity and with the consumption of saturated fat. Here again, modern food processing cannot justly be blamed for plenty nor, in a free society, for providing, side-by-side with margarine high in unsaturated fatty acids, butter high in saturated ones.

In a historical sketch of the impact of modern food technology on nutrition, it is perhaps worth including a few comments on two aspects of what appears to be a wave of public unreason, similar to that which a generation earlier assailed pasteurization.

In 1973, a medical entomologist, B.F. Feingold, claimed that 'salicylate-like' natural components of food, 'low molecular-weight food additives' and artificial colours and flavours, separately and combined, were the cause of what he claimed to be a pathological condition in children which he called 'hyperactivity'(10). Although in later publications Feingold quickly demonstrated his lack of chemical understanding by condemning some foods and withdrawing them from his recommended diets on the basis of chemical compounds they did not contain and including items which he could have been expected from chemical consistency to deplore, and although when, shorn of its academic verbiage, his description of the syndrome of 'hyperactivity' was hard to distinguish from the normal state of naughtiness and high spirits to be expected in the healthy young, Feingold won a large number of disciples, particularly among the better-off classes in the United States, but also in Australia and elsewhere. In view of this and in the light of the ground swell of popular unease about food technology in general, serious studies were made of the Feingold hypothesis(11). As the years roll by and those supporting the thesis linking the supposed disease of 'hyperactivity' with the colouring of foods change their ground, it is hard to avoid the conclusion that the claims as a whole were more in the nature of an emotional response to the problems of living in a wealthy industrial society rather than the interpretation of any serious measurable influence of food technology on nutrition.

A second generalized campaign, widely supported by many people who believe their actions to be based on scientific observations, is that directed against so-called 'junk foods'. Again, it is presumed that the nutritional status of the community is less good than it should be because there is an undue consumption of these products. It is difficult to collect precise evidence upon which the accusation of the unsatisfactory nutrition is based, nor is the definition of the individual items categorized as 'junk foods' always clear and consistent. Individuals are to be found in any society who eat - or, for that matter drink - unwisely but this does not necessarily imply that the individual articles they select are, when used appropriately, unwholesome. Potato crisps, for example, have been designated as 'junk', yet as a snack, they are usefully high in energy value and, furthermore contain 6.3 per cent of protein and 17 mg. of ascorbic acid per 100 g. Another article often attacked as 'junk' is the standardized, fresh-cooked and quickly-served hamburger. The popularity of hamburgers shows that they supply a social need and even a superficial consideration of their composition, as a mixture of bread and meat, frequently supplemented with lettuce and tomato, shows that their ingredients are mainly staple articles of Western diet which have demonstrated their nutritional significance over the centuries.

When I was a boy in the early years of the century, fish and chips, which at that time were cheap and widely eaten by the less fashionable members of the community, were frequently blamed by the intelligentsia for the poor physique of the children of the working classes. Now that fish and chips have become what virtually amount to an expensive delicacy, the nutritional virtues which they always possessed have become generally apparent and it can be seen that their earlier condemnation was not based on scientific evidence but on snobbery. Today, the popular chains of hamburger bars supply the needs of the less-wealthy members of the community and it could be argued that the categorization of hamburgers as 'junk foods' may owe more to snobbery than to a serious consideration of their chemical composition.

If we can allow that responsibility for that most widespread example of malnutrition in Great Britain today, namely obesity, must rest to a major degree on the individual consumer who chooses to eat what he or she does rather than on the manufacturer who makes what he or she eats, the most serious charge which can be brought against those food technologists who so expertly manufacture purified sugar and products made from it is that it is concerned, although less directly than is often assumed, with tooth decay. There are, however, on the market a number of products, ranging from sugar confectionery of various sorts to articles intended to amuse and excite rather than to nourish, in which sugar is a major ingredient. These minor items may also be included within the ambit of 'junk' or 'rubbish' foods. It is, however, sensible to recall that, regardless of its high concentration of sugar, strawberry jam, on which in recent years considerable technical study has been concentrated, is not only an agreeable comestible, but may also encourage the consumption of bread and butter.

Food fulfills three functions, not one. In any consideration of the impact of changing and developing food technology on the nutrition of the British community, it is important to bear in mind that nutrition is only one quality of food. The second is aesthetics. At all levels of nutritional status, even the most stringent when starvation itself has become a threat, the aesthetic quality of food remains important. There may be articles so disgusting that even the deprived will refuse to eat them. While to the food technologist, nutrition and safety are important, more important still is attractiveness. By far the major proportion of all food technologists spend most of their time working to enhance the aesthetic merits of their products. By far the majority of consumers select the food they buy because they like it rather than because they feel that it is particularly nourishing. The best insurance of their obtaining all the nutrients they need lies in their eating a diversity of varied products. For this reason, modern food technology may well be best supporting the well-being of the community by making a wide variety of foodstuffs available throughout the year.

The third criterion of food, interesting to historians and anthropologists, is that it should be fit to eat. The British will not eat the flesh of dogs or horses, nor nowadays, perhaps under the sentimental influence of the Flopsie Bunnies and Bambi, do they select with any enthusiasm meat from rabbits or deer. At the level of wealth enjoyed in Great Britain, these taboos are of little nutritional significance.

Food, health and income

It is generally accepted that during World War II, from 1939 to 1945, the nutritional status of the British public was well maintained. It can now be seen that this happy circumstance was achieved by insuring that enough of a variety of foods was available and, secondly, by looking after the special needs of infants and their mothers. The contribution made by food technology covered a few new developments such as that of dehydrating eggs (not initially a great success) but in the main was concerned with such matter-of-fact problems as the operation of cold stores, the provision of canned meat, the baking of bread, manufacture of butter, margarine and cheese, and the like. Even in those stringent times, however, aesthetics could not be forgotten. One of the lesser known successes of the times was the invention of an egg-substitute called Weiking Eiweiss made from slaughterhouse blood and used by manufacturers to make cake.

But apart from the technological challenges of the war years and the supply of enough food, the satisfactory nutrition of the people was in large measure due to the fact that, since everyone was at work on the war effort, virtually everyone had enough money to buy the food that was equitably distributed on the rations.

During the remainder of the century, it would appear that, so far as the facts are available, the close scrutiny that has been maintained has sufficed to control the use of potentially harmful ingredients or damaging processes in manufactured foods, that the supply and diversity of foods sufficient for a nutritionally adequate diet has been provided, and that the problem of the people obtaining such a diet was more one of insuring an adequate income and the wise expenditure of such than of the application of further virtuosity in food technology.

NOTES

1. Lancet (1977) 1, p. 654.
2. A . Prasad (ed.) Trace Metals in Human Health and Disease (New York, 1976).
3. Proceedings of the Nutrition Society 37 (1978), p. 317.
4. E.P. Cathcart, Nutrition and Dietetics (1928).
5. J.B. Orr, Food, Health and Income (1936).
6. M. Pyke, Food and Society (1968).
7. S. Davidson, R. Passmore, J.F. Brock and A.S. Truswell, Human Nutrition and Dietetics (Edinburgh, 1975).
8. Proceedings of the Royal Society of Medicine 45 (1952), p. 401.
9. Davidson et al, Human Nutrition.
10. Hospital Practice, Oct. 1973, p. 11.
11. Institute of Food Technology, 'Diet and hyperactivity' Nutrition Reviews 34 (1976), p. 151.

3. THE RETAIL AND WHOLESALE MEAT TRADE 1880-1939

RICHARD PERREN

In this survey of the meat trade in Britain for the two generations after 1880 attention will be concentrated on three main themes. The first is an examination of those changes which took place with regard to the areas from which Britain drew its supplies of imported meat - as imported supplies always continued to comprise an important proportion of the total meat consumed in Britain and their importance increased over the whole of this period. The second consideration will be those changes which took place in the organization and conduct of the wholesale and retail meat trades over this period. Thirdly, I will look at the implications which these two preceding features had for the regional pattern of the meat trade in this country.

Table 3.1 shows that the share of imports in the United Kingdom meat supplies increased from something under 30 per cent in 1880 to around 50 per cent by 1923. Thus the meat trade in 1880 was mainly engaged in handling a home-produced article, but by the mid 1920s British meat comprised only half the product that the trade retailed to the public. Unfortunately, it is not possible to continue these comparisons forward on the same basis for the later 1920s and the 1930s. The separation of the Irish Free State in December 1922 meant that country became a foreign state, and the responsibility for its data collection passed to the new government in Dublin. Also no continuous estimates of total meat consumption for the United Kingdom were published after 1924(1). Estimates of home-produced output were published for England and Wales in the annual Agricultural Statistics(2), and for Scotland up to 1930(3). Therefore, the basis of the home-produced component of the three later estimates in Table 3.1 is uncertain but they probably use these sources with some sort of allowance being made for Northern Ireland. However, these figures from John Boyd Orr's survey(4) and Forrest Capie's article(5) do provide sufficient grounds for believing that the reliance on imported meat increased after 1923. To some extent this would be expected as the separation of Ireland meant animals imported from there directly for slaughter were now classed as foreign meat. The decline in the share of imported meats after 1932 is mostly explained by the relative and absolute fall in imported pig-meat, although there was some relative decline in the share of imported beef and veal against home-produced as well. But although the United Kingdom market was made less attractive to overseas suppliers by various measures to regulate imports after 1931, their share still remained at about 54 per cent for the later 1930s which was something of a fall from the high point of 61.8 per cent in 1931(6).

The increase in the proportion of imported meat permitted a rise in consumption per head. Before the First War the high point was 130 lbs per head in 1900-09; thereafter it fell slightly. The reason for this was that there was further pressure on supply as the population in some of the former exporting countries(7) - in particular the United States - rose to absorb most of their export surplus. The fact that this fall in consumption was due to supply constraints is reinforced by the modest rise in animal product prices, which had fallen for the 1880s and early 1890s after 1896(8). The shortage of shipping space in the First War also meant some pressure on supply, and so was responsible for the fall per head between 1915 and 1919. There was no immediate recovery in supplies on the return to peace; for one thing United Kingdom herds had been drastically reduced in the latter stages of the war, when strategic needs dictated greater concentration in corn growing at the expense of livestock farming(9). To some extent, the increase per head in consumption after 1924 is a statistical mirage. Traditionally, meat consumption in Ireland had always been lower than the rest of the United Kingdom and in fact she was a net exporter to Great Britain. Therefore, the removal of Ireland from the United Kingdom figures was bound to produce an apparent rise in consumption per head for the remaining population. But the maintenance of consumption per head well

Table 3.1: Annual average meat supply for the United Kingdom

	3.1.1 Beef and Veal			3.1.2 Mutton and Lamb		
	Home pro- duction	Net imports	Proportion of home to total supplies	Home pro- duction	Net imports	Proportion of home to total supplies
	(000 tons)	(000 tons)	(%)	(000 tons)	(000 tons)	(%)
1880-89	690	162	81.0	363	54	87.0
1890-99	742	326	69.5	393	143	73.3
1900-09	749	429	63.6	303	212	58.8
1910-14	781	484	61.7	311	269	53.6
1915-19	751	451	62.4	267	185	59.0
1920-23	694	593	53.9	223	308	42.0
1924-28	624	673	48.1	221	270	46.0
1929-32	592	729	44.8	213	332	39.1
1933-36	633	665	48.8	224	338	39.9
1936-39	675	733	47.9	235	353	40.0

Sources:

1980-99   R. Perren, The Meat Trade in Britain 1840-1914 (1978), p.3.

1900-23   First Report Royal Commission on Food Prices Parliamentary Papers 1924-25 XIII, p. 162.

1924-28   J.B. Orr, Food Health and Income (1936), Appendix III.

1929-39   Home Production: F. Capie, 'Australian and New Zealand Competition in the British Market, 1920-39', Australian Economic History Review Vol. XVIII (1978), p. 62. Net Imports: United Kingdom Annual Statement of Trade, Tables of Retained Imports.

Table 3.1: (Contd.)

3.1.3		Pig Meat	3.1.4	Total Consumption	
Home production	Net imports	Proportion of home to total supplies	All kinds of meat	Proportion of home to total supplies	Consumption per head
(000 tons)	(000 tons)	(%)	(000 tons)	(%)	(lbs)
253	222	53.3	1,775	73.6	110.8
270	313	46.3	2,209	63.6	126.6
403	369	52.2	2,489	58.4	130.3
393	317	55.4	2,575	57.7	126.9
301	455	39.3	2,441	54.0	122.6
361	413	46.6	2,592	49.3	123.2
318	490	39.3	2,596	44.8	128.6
327	578	36.1	2,777	40.8	135.3
416	482	46.3	2,765	46.0	132.4
454	455	49.9	2,909	46.9	137.2

Note 1:   All Ireland is included until 1924 after which the Irish Free State is excluded.

2:   Small quantities of undifferentiated imported meat are included within the Total Consumption column.

above 130 lbs for the 1930s was a reflection of the abundant supply of primary products in that decade, and a benefit to the consumer. It was the failure of the domestic producer to hold his share of the home market after 1920 which gave rise to a number of investigations which provide us with much of our information on the meat trade after the First World War - the Marketing Reports carried out by the Ministry of Agriculture. Although these surveys were aimed at discovering ways of assisting the British farmer it is doubtful whether they provided him much practical help. Their suggestions came in two categories: firstly, greater concentration on the production of a high quality product, and secondly, schemes for marking home-produced meat so that the consumer could always positively select the home-produced article. But at the same time these reports contained comprehensive surveys of the scope, structure and organization of the whole imported and domestic meat trade in Britain.

The growth of imports

In 1880 the most important sources of imported meat were North America and Europe. North America was principally the United States which supplied pig-meat and beef. Certainly United States pig-meat at this time was not a high quality product. It was very fatty and was preserved for the voyage across the Atlantic by packing it aboard ship in layers of salt. Beef at that time was sent partly on the hoof in the transatlantic cattle ships and also as salted beef. A very small quantity was also sent under conditions of refrigeration - but at that time this trade was merely in its infancy. European meat came in as livestock and also as fresh dead meat - the problem of distance did not require importers to resort to salting.

After 1880 the really big growth in imported supplies of beef came from North America and after 1900 from South America. In the case of sheep and mutton, New Zealand and Australia were, and remained, the main suppliers with the development of the frozen meat trade from those countries after 1882(10). Although in 1880 the main source of imported beef was North America, by 1900 its importance had started to decline. The centre of gravity of the international beef trade was moving southwards(11). By the First World War the United States had ceased to be a serious contributor of

our supplies of chilled beef - in the 1880s the
United States supplied approximately 800,000 cwt
of chilled beef annually; in 1913 it supplied 1,462
cwt - the American export trade had been transferred to the Argentine. In the 1920s the latter country and Uruguay constituted the only area which
was a large exporter of chilled beef(12). But
the chilled beef trade had been pioneered from
the United States by firms from that country, and
they did not relinquish their control over this
trade because the continent·from which it was supplied changed. Even before the First World War
American firms were strongly entrenched in the
conduct of the export of beef from the River Plate
to this country(13). Whereas the imported beef
trade had been subject to marked geographical
shifts over this period, the trade in imported
mutton and lamb underwent no such change. The
growth of the frozen mutton trade from New Zealand
and to a lesser extent from Australia began soon
after 1880, and by the First World War New Zealand
was the major overseas producer, followed by Australia. This position remained the same in the
1920s, with New Zealand predominantly the country
of first-grade mutton and lamb, and Australia generally supplying a rather more inferior product.
Another contrast between the imported beef and
mutton trade is that the former were predominantly
chilled carcasses and the latter were predominantly
frozen.
      Over the whole of this period the only area
of the meat supply in which the European influence
was reinforced was with regard to pig-meat. In
1880 when Britain was almost entirely dependent
upon the United States for its imports of bacon
and ham, over 90 per cent came from across the
Atlantic. After 1880, the dependence of this country on American supplies diminished with the growth
of imports from Canada, Denmark and, later, Sweden
and Russia. By 1913 just under 45 per cent of
the United Kingdom's imports of bacon and hams
came from the United States. The most important
of these new suppliers was Denmark. Only to a
slight extent did Danish bacon actually displace
the American - because Danish bacon which was a
high quality, mild cured, lean bacon. Thus the
Danes created and supplied a new and important
demand in the British market. In contrast to the
imported bacon and ham trade, that in imported
fresh pork, because of problems of storage and
preservation, was very small. This product was

51

traditionally a European one and the trade had existed before the 1880s. By 1925, out of a total quantity of pig-meat of over 10 million hundred-weights imported, three-quarters was accounted for by bacon alone(14). The First World War temporarily diverted supplies from Denmark to Germany, but on the resumption of peace the trade in imported bacon settled down largely along the lines it had assumed before the war.

The structure of the meat trade

The changes which increased dependence on overseas sources of supply imposed on the British meat trade were themselves quite considerable. A whole network of traders was established after 1880 to handle imported meat. This meant the entry of new firms into the trade; wholesaling organizations that sold only foreign meat but later sold home and foreign in the same shop. Again, because the individual quantities that arrived in this country were very large by comparison with the amounts that the British meat producer released onto the market, quite different methods of distribution were required to ensure a smooth distribution from dock to dinner-table. Indeed, it is quite plausible to argue that without the growing reliance on imported meat, the influence of the large-scale marketing firm in this industry would have been very much weaker. This is because it was in the imported meat trade that the large firm made its influence felt first. In the early 1880s the first retail firm in Britain with over 100 butchers' shops was John Bell & Sons of Glasgow who, although they were a relatively old-established Scottish business dating back to 1827, were by that time involved in the sale of North American meat in Britain. Although the importers of meat soon extended their activities into the retail trade, by 1900 over 88 per cent of meat sales were by small retail firms - most of these the single-shop variety(15).

The growth of the large multiple company in the meat industry was regarded as a sinister phenomenon, both before and after the First War(16). Before 1914 attention was directed towards the American "trust" companies, who extended their operations into the United Kingdom from around 1891 onwards, when the American firm of Swift first purchased a store in the Central Markets of Smithfield. By 1900 the transatlantic beef and cattle trade was controlled by the firms Armour and Company, Swift and Company, and Morris and Company. After 1902, as imports of North American beef into Britain started to diminish, the North American firms turned their attention to obtaining an important share of the South American beef trade. This move was an insurance by the North American firms against the time when the USA would have no surplus of meat available for export. By 1913 North American firms held a dominant share of the export of beef from South America to the United Kingdom. However their position in this trade was challenged after the First World War by the growth of the Vestey family organization - the Union Cold Storage Company. This firm, founded in 1897 with a capital of £50,000, and one cold storage establishment, had by the mid-1920s a paid-up share capital of nearly £9,000,000, and was allied to a dozen subsidiary companies operating in the Argentine as well as the Australian trade and owned about a third of Britain's cold storage facilities. However, although the entry of this British-owned firm into the imported meat trade was an insurance against complete American domination, the size of this firm was viewed with some alarm in Britain. It was alleged that the company presented a threat to the normal practices of retail competition. It was also argued that any agreement between the American firms and Vestey's could establish a virtual monopoly in our imported beef supplies - something which some saw as fraught with great danger to the consuming public of the country(17)!

These fears were widely expressed by the smaller British meat trader in the years after the First World War. In the 1920s there was some dispute as to whether the consumption of meat had been rising or falling since the war. Statistics of imports and home production certainly pointed to an increase in consumption since 1918. On the other hand retail traders giving evidence to the Royal Commission on Food Prices which reported in 1925 argued that consumption had decreased since 1913. The president of the National Federation of Meat Traders' Association stated that in his experience far less was eaten in middle-class households, and a representative of the Scottish Federation of Meat Traders' Association put the average reduction in Scotland at one-third. A co-operative witness supported the view that consumption per family was less, but attributed this largely to the smaller size of families. It seems that the reason for this apparent decrease was accounted for in many places by an increase in the number of butchers' shops. The population of the British Isles increased from 45.7 million in 1913 to 47.8 million in 1923, or approximately 4.5 per cent in ten years(18). The Linlithgow Committee's report on meat in 1923 calculated, from samples of 100 towns in England and Wales and 30 towns in Scotland that the number of shops had increased by 7.5 per cent and by 15 per cent respectively between 1913 and 1923(19). As aggregate consumption in the 1920s was only around 2 per cent greater than it had been in the years immediately before the First War, it was inevitable that the increased number of retail outlets meant that each outlet was handling a reduced volume of sales. But it was the independent butcher who was hardest hit by this development. Jefferys presents estimates of the shares of different types of retailer in the total sales of meat from 1900. Then co-operative societies and multiple shops accounted for between 7.5 per cent and 12 per cent of meat sold; by 1925 the two had increased their share to between 13 per cent and 18 per cent(20).

One fear that was expressed by certain classes of retail butchers before the war was the fear that the growth of the large multiple shop companies would reduce competition. However there is little evidence that the retail trade was subject to substantially less competition in the 1920s than it had been at any earlier date. One survey, covering the years between 1921 and 1931, for twelve towns in England shows that the relative number of butchers' shops rose, although the same study does indicate a fall from 1901 to 1921(21). Competition existed between departmental stores, co-operative societies, multiple companies, and the traditional individual trader. There was no possibility of agreement among retailers to keep up prices, and neither the National Federation, the Scottish Federation, nor local associations of butchers throughout the country ever attempted to give directions as to the prices their members should charge. Sometimes retail butchers in a district might form an association for the purpose of buying livestock at local markets. But there was no possibility of having such an organization for the purpose of selling to the public; in any case even in the livestock market their buyer would be acting in competition with those from surrounding towns and villages.

In the 1920s there was a reduction in the number of shops in the hands of multiple shop companies. This is accounted for by the amalgamation of several large shop companies in the hands of the Union Cold Storage Company. By the middle 1920s this organization operated 2,356 retail shops which had formerly belonged to three companies, Eastmans Limited, The British and Argentine Company, The Argenta Meat Company, as well as a number of other companies and firms. There was considerable variation between the prices charged in the Union Cold Storage Company's shops in different parts of the country, and the managers there were left considerable discretion in fixing prices to meet competition between the branches themselves as there was when they were owned by separate companies. Moreover, the policy of the Union Cold Storage Company was to close down the less profitable shops, with the result that in many places the number of competing multiple shops was less than it was when they were under separate control before the First World War(22).

Some members of the public believed that there was less competition between retailers than before 1914. Among the factors suggested were the diminution in a number of butchers' stores and barrows; the more hygienic and expensive type of shop which the public were demanding, and the larger capital which was required to start a new business. The competition brought about by the growth of co-operative butchery departments was not so effective as it might otherwise have been owing to their general practice in most cases in making a net profit of about 10 per cent and thus distributing a dividend of 2s. in the pound. It was thought that co-operative societies were of little assistance in keeping down prices, at any rate in those districts where good dividend was more popular with the members than low prices(23).

Therefore, all these developments - the entry of more firms into the trade after the War; the rationalization movement among large retailers; the aggressive pursuit of the 10 per cent dividend by co-operative societies' butchers perhaps indicate that life was harder for the independent retailer. Under the protected conditions of wartime bankruptcies were rare, but climbed sharply after 1921. The small retailers were not really frightened by the prospect of less competition but by the increase of a different kind of competition.

They feared the market power of the big retailing firms and were conscious of their own weakness vis-a-vis such giants as Vestey's Dewhurst chain.

Consumer preferences

The implications of some of these changes for the trade on a regional level were quite clear. For instance, because they required a large volume of sales, the importing firms were more likely to be found in the large towns and cities than the villages. This was noticeable before 1914 and right through this period. From this it also follows that the urban population of Britain ate a higher proportion of imported meat than did the inhabitants of smaller towns and rural dwellers. In 1907 80 per cent of the meat sold in Dundee, 90 per cent of that sold in Newcastle and almost 100 per cent of that sold in Norwich was home-produced, whereas 50 per cent of Manchester's meat was foreign and in London over 80 per cent of meat sold at Smithfield was foreign(24). This was partly a function of size of market but it is also explained by the proximity to the ports. London and Liverpool were the two chief ports receiving imported meat over the whole 50 years and it was natural that their markets were supplied first, and any which they could not absorb was then railed to other places. However, these two ports did not have an absolute monopoly of meat imports. For instance, the principal ports through which frozen mutton and lamb and chilled and frozen beef entered Great Britain in the 1920s were London, Liverpool, Southampton, Manchester, Hull, Avonmouth, Newcastle and Glasgow. Chilled imports were however confined to the first three. Before the First World War Liverpool had been the business centre of the imported meat trade, owing to its convenient situation for North Atlantic shipments, and London remained the finance centre. With the decline of the North American trade this position changed, and the trade tended to focus on London. By the 1920s it was noticed there were slight differences in the class of goods shipped to each port - Glasgow took large quantities of boneless beef, but was not a great importer of mutton. (Perhaps this reflects the higher production and consumption of beef in Scotland than of mutton.) In Liverpool and generally in the north of England - excepting perhaps Newcastle-on-Tyne - light carcasses and quarters were preferred, even if the quality was not particularly good. In London, heavier weights were taken, which was convenient for importers, as they shipped their lighter weights to Liverpool and other outports, and brought their heavier first-class goods received in those ports into London. However, we should not make too much of these differences.

Theoretically, the meat ports were admirably placed for dealing with and distributing the meat each received to the centres of population that surrounded them. Enquiries at the time however showed that although each of the meat ports was regularly used, to some extent, for the distribution of supplies in its own area, each also contributed to the areas of the others. From Newcastle, for example, apart from railing meat to centres of consumption within its own area, meat was also railed to Edinburgh and Glasgow, Lancashire (including Manchester and Liverpool), South Yorkshire, the Midlands, and occasionally even to London; meat was received - in the order of tonnage - from Liverpool, Hull, Manchester and Glasgow. Hull sent supplies to Lancashire, Yorkshire, the Midlands and London, and received meat from London, Manchester, Liverpool and Newcastle. The persistence of this system - at first sight seeming to be wasteful - was due in the main to two factors. Firstly, each importing firm distributed its own meat without reference to the others, and met its orders from any supplies which it had available at any port. It was natural, therefore, that cross-railing should occur where so many firms had organizations which served the same area. Secondly, there was the difficulty of arranging regular freight to any but the two chief ports - London and Liverpool; a shipping company may have insisted upon a minimum tonnage before a ship was sent to an outport, and such a minimum may have been beyond the local requirements of the importer. Therefore it was cheaper to bring the meat to London or Liverpool and then to rail the exact requirements to the outport districts than to shop supplies directly there at the cost of excessive freight(25).

One feature which was noticed by the trade over the whole of this time, and which applied both to domestically-produced and imported meat was the demand for lighter carcasses. This can be accounted for by the fact that the British housewife preferred to purchase smaller joints in 1930 than she did in 1880. We can see this in all branches of the meat trade, both foreign and domestic and it applies to all types of meat - mutton and lamb, beef, pork and bacon. For instance, the British demand for frozen mutton when it first appeared on the market was for relatively heavy carcasses. In 1887 the most favoured weight at Smithfield was a 64 lb carcass, but by 1910 it had fallen to a carcass that weighed between 48 and 52 lbs(26). This preference was also reflected in price. In the 1920s second-grade imported New Zealand lambs of a desirable weight - from about 24 to 34 lbs - frequently commanded a better price and met a readier sale than first-grade from 36 to 42 lbs(27). By the 1920s heavy mutton - that is from carcasses of above 60 lbs - was only in demand for certain special purposes, such as for contracts for the fighting services, and, except in times of great shortage, it was only saleable at very low prices on the civilian market. But it must be emphasized that such popularity among consumers was not necessarily a complete reflection of quality. The Report on the Marketing of Sheep, Mutton and Lamb felt that 'It cannot be too strongly emphasized that carcass weight is a price determinant equal in importance to quality and quite independent of it'(28). It also depended on such things as the type of animal from which the carcass came - for instance whether, ewe, or maiden ewe - and its age at slaughter. It was argued, in explaining this preference for lighter carcasses, that the English working classes wanted more variety on their table, and that in the case of this meat, the English housewife was less bothered to prepare dishes from cold mutton. Meat traders complained that public taste was more difficult to cater for than before the war. Smaller joints were demanded and there was greater difficulty in disposing of the cheaper cuts. It was stated that the public exercised more discrimination as to what they purchased. The better cuts of imported meat were preferred to inferior qualities of home-killed. One view expressed was that the decline in housing accommodation as a result of the war meant that many housewives had inferior cooking facilities. It was argued that this meant that there was a falling off in the demand for stewing meat. The same cause was said to be responsible for an increase in the popularity of tinned foods(29). In the case of the pork and bacon trade there was certainly a demand for lighter-weight pork carcasses. However, the position here is complicated by the greatly differing demands of the different sections of these trades. In general, specialised bacon curers wanted a heavier pig than most family butchers. But the weight required varied between different groups of curers. Ayrshire rolled bacon producers wanted a carcass between 140 to 170 lbs(30). The regional pattern of demand also varied. In the mining districts of Lancashire there was a demand for fat pork from heavy pigs, presumably because the high energy value of this meat was appreciated by those engaged in heavy manual work, but fat pork was reputedly disliked by factory workers. Also in the coastal towns of the county during the summer months there was a heavy demand for small lean porkers to feed the holiday visitors(31). But one feature of the retail trade which was noticeable in the interwar years was the rapidly increasing extent to which bacon was sold in the form of rashers instead of as cuts, as was more common before the First War. In fact in large cities and industrial areas generally, it was very rarely that whole cuts of bacon were sold retail at all by the 1920s. This revolution in the trade was brought about by the introduction of slicing machines, which came to form part of the equipment of every modern shop. In some districts, slicing machines were also fitted up in grocers' vans which went from house to house calling for orders and delivering the goods there and then. Some country retailers, who were not equipped with the mechanical slicer, sometimes bought their supplies ready sliced from the wholesaler; so that, even in agricultural districts, the practice of selling bacon by the piece was rapidly giving way to the sale of rashers. Again, this tendency - buying bacon in the form of rashers - made it difficult for the consumer to identify the branding or marking of the product unless the rashering was done in his or her presence, or, they were able to view the piece before it was sliced(32).

Before the First World War, home and imported supplies were usually handled separately, right through the whole network of distribution up to the table of the consumer. There was a trickle from the imported stream into butchers' shops which also sold home-killed, but as a rule the sale of imported meat was confined to retail establishments which specialized in that trade. To obtain imported meat therefore, the ordinary consumer had to buy from a shop which traded in nothing else, and owing to the prejudice against imported supplies, often incurred some social stigma in doing so. In 1914 there were many thousands of people in the country who had never knowingly tasted imported beef, and on thousands of butchers' counters it had never found a place. By the middle of the 1920s this position had entirely changed; people who before the war never ate imported meat now ate nothing else, and though there were still many retailers who confined their trade to fresh-killed meat, yet the majority included imported meat in their buying, and many went over entirely to the imported meat trade. It was common to find butchers, even with a high-class family trade, displaying a notice to the effect that all meat sold in their establishment was foreign unless otherwise stated. The offering for sale of home and imported meat, side by side, in the same shop, made the alternative an immediate one, and imported meat had selling opportunities which were unknown and undreamt of before the First War(33).

To some extent it was a trade which did not escape official scrutiny. Under the sale of food order of 1921 it was forbidden to expose for retail sale any imported meat unless this meat bore a label with the word 'Imported' or words disclosing the country of origin, or unless a notice was exhibited in a conspicuous position indicating that only imported meat was on sale in that shop. Despite the fact that in some parts of the country serious efforts were made to enforce the provisions of this order, in general it appeared to be a dead letter. One reaction in the later 1920s was the passing of the Agricultural Produce (Grading and Marking) Acts of 1928 and 1929, which permitted home producers to participate in voluntary schemes to sell a standardized product under a National Mark. However, such schemes did not find much popularity with British farmers, possibly because of the very wide range of qualities for domestically-produced meat and the high percentage of low quality(34). The motive behind this legislation was the allegation that imported meat was substituted as home-produced which allowed it to command the higher price which home-produced meat fetched. But for such a practice to be possible the two meats had to be close to each other in quality, or else the customer particularly naive and easily duped. The substitution of imported for home-produced had been alleged before 1914(35), and such allegations do not seem to have diminished much after.

One study of consumer preferences for the interwar period concludes that foreign and home-produced meat did not in fact compete directly and that the two trades ran separate courses. Imported refrigerated meat was not considered superior, or even equal, to the fresh home-produced article(36). But it must also be remembered that the British farmer was vociferous in his complaints throughout most of these years. Ideally, he would have liked protection against all agricultural imports, not just, or particularly, meat. This was a plain impossibility. But the foregoing legislation and marketing schemes cost politicians nothing in terms of higher food prices or lost votes. Such pieces of window-dressing could also be represented as attempts to protect home producers from 'unfair competition' - whatever that might have meant - as well as guarding the consumer from inaccurate product descriptions. There does appear to have been some surprising ignorance about products on the part of the public. In the 1920s a leading member of the imported mutton trade observed that many of the housewives of London, who bought Canterbury lamb, imagined that they were buying lamb of Kentish origin(37)! But the deception applied also to different qualities within the imported meat trade. For example, many consumers were not aware that much of the imported lamb and mutton on the English market was of South American and not of Empire origin. That substitution of one kind of imported lamb for another took place was clearly shown by the frequent prosecutions instigated by the representative of the New Zealand meat producers board, where an inferior foreign article had been sold as Canterbury or New Zealand lamb(38). One result of substitution, so far as the home-killed trade was concerned, is that consumers often preferred definitely to order imported rather than home-killed meat, owing to the uncertainty as to what would otherwise be supplied at the price of the home-killed article.

NOTES

1. Imperial Economic Committee on Marketing and Preparing for Market of Foodstuffs; Second Report - Meat, Parliamentary Papers 1924-25 XIII, pp. 5-6.
2. Ministry of Agriculture and Fisheries,

Agricultural Statistics England and Wales. In addition estimates of agricultural output were made in the censuses of production for 1925 and 1930: see The Agricultural Output of England and Wales 1925 Parliamentary Papers 1927 XXV; The Agricultural Output of England and Wales 1930-31 Parliamentary Papers 1933-34 XXVI. Also, the Ministry's Reports on Marketing contain some estimates of meat production in Britain up to the various dates they were written: in particular, see Report on the Marketing of Pigs (Economic Series, No.12) 1926 p. 98; Report on the Marketing of Cattle and Beef (Economic Series, No. 20) 1929 p. 153; Report on the Marketing of Sheep, Mutton and Lamb (Economic Series, No. 29) 1931, p. 174.

3.   Board of Agriculture for Scotland, The Agricultural Output of Scotland 1929 Parliamentary Papers 1928-29 V, p. 34; The Agricultural Output of Scotland 1930 Parliamentary Papers, 1933-34 XXVI, p. 26.

4.   Orr's survey used estimates for 1924-28 made by Sir Alfred Flux, 'Our Food Supply before and after the War', Journal of the Royal Statistical Society Vol. 93 (1930), pp. 538-56, and for 1924-27 by A.E. Feaveryear, 'The National Expenditure, 1932', Economic Journal Vol. 43 (1934), pp. 34-47. The 1934 estimates were made by the Market Supply Committee established by the Ministry of Agriculture and Fisheries, with Feaveryear's assistance. Ibid., pp. 10-11, 14.

5.   See F. Capie, 'Australian and New Zealand Competition in the British Market, 1920-39', Australian Economic History Review Vol. XVIII (1978), pp. 46-62. Capie's article contains annual estimates of home-produced and imported meats from 1920 to 1939. These are substantially in agreement with Boyd Orr's for the years when the two overlap (i.e., 1924-28, 1934). However, Capie adopts a stricter definition of meat than the one used in Table 3.1 because he excludes edible offal from his totals; see p. 46, footnote 1. An allowance has been made for this in Table 3.1 by adding 10 per cent to Capie's home-produced beef, veal, mutton and lamb totals and 5 per cent to his home-produced pig-meat totals. As offal is also excluded from his estimates of imports these have been re-calculated

directly from the United Kingdom Annual Statement of Trade for 1929-39. Neither the inclusion nor exclusion of offals substantially alters the market shares of imported and home-produced.

6. K.A.H. Murray, Agriculture (1955), pp. 29-31. Capie, A.Ec. H.R. Vol. XVIII pp. 53, 62.
7. This change was foreseen by R.H. Hooker, 'The Meat Supply of the United Kingdom' J.R.S.S. Vol. 72 (1909), pp. 310, 350-352.
8. B.R. Mitchell and P. Deane, Abstract of British Historical Statistics (1962), pp. 472-3, 474-5.
9. E.H. Whetham, The Agrarian History of England & Wales, Volume VIII 1914-39 (1978), pp. 124-6.
10. J.T.Critchell and J. Raymond, A History of the Frozen Meat Trade (1912). Imperial Economic Committee, Mutton and Lamb Survey (1935), pp. 148-159.
11. Ministry of Agriculture and Fisheries, Report on the Trade in Refrigerated Beef, Mutton and Lamb (Economic Series, No. 6) (1925), pp. 7-8.
12. R. Perren, 'The North American Beef and Cattle Trade with Britain, 1870-1914', Economic History Review 2nd series Vol. XXIV (1971), p. 432. Intelligence Branch of the Imperial Economic Committee, Cattle and Beef Survey (1934), pp. 189-90.
13. Report of Inter-Departmental Committee on Meat Supplies Parliamentary Papers 1919 XV, p.9.
14. Ministry of Agriculture and Fisheries, Report on the Pork and Bacon Trades (Economic Series No. 17) (1928), pp. 10-12; Report on the Marketing of Pigs (Economic Series, No. 12) (1926), pp. 2-9.
15. J.B. Jeffreys, Retail Trading in Britain, 1850-1950 (Economic and Social Studies, No.13) (Cambridge, 1954), pp. 187, 201.
16. Inter-Departmental Committee on Combinations in the Meat Trade Parliamentary Papers 1909 XV; Standing Committee on Trusts - Interim Report on Meat Parliamentary Papers 1920 XXIII; Report on Refrigerated Beef, Mutton and Lamb, pp. 51-3.
17. First Report Royal Commission on Food Prices Parliamentary Papers 1924-25 XIII, paras. 235, 295.

18. First Report Royal Commission on Food Prices,
    p. 78.
19. Ministry of Agriculture and Fisheries, Depart-
    mental Committee on Distribution and Prices
    of Agricultural Produce - Interim Report on
    Meat, Poultry and Eggs Cmd. 1927 (1923), pp.
    173-176.
20. Jefferys, Retail Trading, p. 201.
21. P. Ford, 'Decentralization and Changes in
    the Number of Shops', Economic Journal Vol.
    46 (1935), p. 360.
22. Jefferys, Retail Trading, pp. 192-3, 194; First
    Report Royal Commission on Food Prices, pp.
    97-8.
23. First Report Royal Commission on Food Prices,
    p. 98.
24. R. Perren, Ec.H.R. Vol. XXIV p. 440.
25. Report on Refrigerated Beef, Mutton and Lamb,
    pp. 32-6.
26. Critchell and Raymond, Frozen Meat Trade,
    p. 107 (But the Imperial Economic Committee
    on Marketing Second Report - Meat, p. 17,
    reported that 'In the case of mutton the most
    desirable weights range from 50 to 60 lb').
27. Report on the Trade in Refrigerated Beef,
    Mutton and Lamb, p. 18.
28. Report on the Marketing of Sheep, Mutton and
    Lamb, p. 156.
29. First Report Royal Commission on Food Prices,
    pp. 79-80.
30. Report on the Marketing of Pigs, pp. 31-6.
31. V. Liversage, 'The Lancashire Pig Trade',
    Journal of the Ministry of Agriculture Vol.
    XXXVI (1929), p. 250.
32. Report on the Pork and Bacon Trades, pp. 144-
    6.
33. Report on Refrigerated Beef, Mutton and Lamb,
    p. 46.
34. Ministry of Agriculture and Fisheries and
    the Scottish Office, Report of the Second
    Inter-Departmental Committee on the Grading
    and Marking of Beef Cmd. 4047 (1932); J.Hunt-
    er Smith and H.W. Gardner, 'Super-English
    or Baby Beef', Jnl. Min. Ag. Vol. XXXV (1928)
    p. 730.
35. 'The Sale of Foreign Meat as British', The
    Parish Councillor Vol. II (1896), pp. 167,
    183, 199. Select Committee on Agricultural
    Produce (Marks) Bill Parliamentary Papers
    1897 VIII.
36. Capie, 'Consumer Preference; Meat in England

and Wales, 1920-1938', Bulletin of Economic Research Vol. 28 (1976), pp. 87-90.

37. Report on the Marketing of Sheep, Mutton and Lamb.

38. Ibid.

4. THE DEMAND FOR MEAT IN ENGLAND AND WALES BETWEEN THE TWO WORLD WARS

FORREST CAPIE

For much of the twentieth century, meat, broadly defined and in value terms, has been the world's second largest internationally traded commodity. In the inter-war years Britain was the world's biggest market for the product and meat was Britain's largest single import(1). It is not surprising therefore that much attention has been given to the supply of meat to the British consumer(2). Against this analysis of the demand for meat has been badly neglected, in spite of the considerable interest that lies in knowing more about the pattern of consumer's preference for such an important item in the family budget(3). There are several reasons why an examination of the demand for meat in the inter-war years can be of value. Firstly there is the obvious one of shedding some light on living standards in the period. Associated with this is the interest that lies in identifying the factors important in determining demand. There is also the possibility in demand analysis of showing the extent of price and income responsiveness and the degree of substitutability between varieties of the product. The latter in turn may suggest which policies should have proved most effective in, for example, the raising of prices or the promotion of the home produced variety at the expense of the imported one.

This article shows that in general price elasticities for imported meats were higher than those for home produced meats. Income elasticities generally conformed to theoretical expectations in both size and magnitude though an exception was found in New Zealand lamb. And substitution elasticities tended to support the other results. Whilst an examination of the contemporary evidence

66

on meat consumption is full of difficulties of
interpretation some of it does seem to suggest
that as income increased so too did total meat
consumption but this was largely accounted for
by the increased variety of meats within
the total(4). A simple correlation of income with
specific types of meat was not always positive.

Sources and methods

There are two main sources for the quantities
of meats: The Trade and Navigation Accounts for
the imported product(5) and the Ministry of Agriculture's publications for the domestic product(6).
Imports in the Accounts are given according to
the appropriate preservation category (fresh,chill-
ed, frozen, salted, etc.) and further sub-divided
by cut (hindquarters, forequarters, boneless,
tongues, offal etc.). A collation was made of
the principal cuts in each preservation category
excluding all lesser types such as tongues and
kidneys. When therefore reference is made to Argentine beef, it is the principal variety of that
product, namely chilled hindquarters that is being
discussed. Similarly New Zealand lamb is made
up of the main cuts of New Zealand frozen lamb
and so on. This was done primarily because of
prices available and also to come closer to the
retail description of meats. Production statistics
for the domestically produced item have been provided in various forms by the Ministry of Agriculture and Fisheries, and while not always ideal
for the purpose, it was possible to build up an
annual series for the period, of the major types
of meat. There are then quantities of British,
Australian, Argentinian and New Zealand lamb, mutton and beef; the last item usually included the
insignificant quantities of veal. In other words
in this analysis it is possible to test twelve
varieties of meat; and these varieties made up
by far the greatest proportion of all meat consumed
in Britain.
The Ministry of Agriculture also provided
excellent series on prices. These are available
in monthly form as well as annual, though it was
the latter that were of use for matching with the
annual quantity data. In some instances no matching price and quantity figures were available and
where this was the case an a priori close substitute's price was used as surrogate. For example,
an average price for British beef was not available

but individual prices for English long sides, English short sides etc. were, whereas the quantities available were for British beef as a whole. Each of the beef prices was used in turn as a proxy for the average.

The income series used was net national income at current prices deflated by the cost-of-living index, and population figures are as given in Stone(7).

The aim of the demand analysis is to estimate parameters such as own-price elasticities and the estimation is carried out by multiple regression analysis on time series data for 1920-1938. Some have argued that the demand for a perishable agricultural commodity is different from that of an industrial product, the direction of causation being reversed, current price being influenced by the clearing of the market, and for this reason single regression equations were estimated in which price was expressed as a function of quantity coming on to the market. (This procedure is not strictly necessary, very similar results being obtained when the demand function is estimated in conventional form.) No account was taken of stocks in view of the perishable nature of the product and the fact that even for the frozen variety of the product (i.e. the most easily kept), stocks were infinitessimal. Many studies have proceeded in this manner, regarding supply as exogenously determined(8). The fact that Britain was the major world market for this product and that there were few opportunities open to foreign suppliers like Australia and New Zealand for diverting exports elsewhere, strengthens this point.

The main question to be settled is, how much was consumption affected by price and the price of other meats or other foods, and how much by income.

The approach to demand is to use a single equation in which it is argued the correct identifying variables are income, price, and prices of other goods. Population is taken account of by using per capita data. Logging the variables provides the proportionate change in each and a simple transformation produces the desired elasticities(9). These parameters are useful for grouping and arranging the varieties according to the degree of responsiveness to price and income and substitutability. The procedure followed in each case was first to regress price on quantity for each product and then to introduce the quantities of other meats

into the equations and finally to observe the influence of income. The results presented here,
together with some discussion, are simply a selection from the total.

Elasticities

Table 4.1 provides a sample of the results
which are typical of the total obtained and the
general comments which might be made are that:
the signs and magnitudes of the various elasticities
are very largely in agreement with theoretical
expectations (the main exception in the results
being one negative income elasticity to which I
shall return later); a good level of explanation
is frequently obtained; autocorrelation was a problem on occasions, leading to the rejection of some
of the equations. The results show that, for example, the direct price elasticity for Australian
frozen lamb was much greater than that for British
lamb and the suggestion here is that the former
product was more sensitive to price movement –
perhaps through having more substitutes than the
British variety. Argentine frozen lamb was found
to be comparable with Australian while New Zealand
lamb fell between these two and the British, though
closer to the latter. Results of this kind suggesting a different market for these varieties are
supported by contemporary views such as the following: 'Possibly the English and the import trades
run separate courses in detail, and are devoted
each to its own consuming class '(10).

Following the analysis for the whole period
1920-1938, the period was split into two sub-periods
1920-30 and 1928-38, keeping, in both cases, a
sample size of eleven observations – hence the
overlap. This was done in order to see if there
were any significant differences between the 1920s
and the 1930s, or to see if there were some identi-
fiable structural change in the period. The results
obtained were always in doubt. The small sample
reduced our confidence, though it must be said
that the results were everywhere as good as those
obtained for the period as a whole. For example
for British lamb the equations are similar for
both sub-periods, and close direct price elasticity
estimates were obtained. The income coefficient
also seems to be in agreement with the aggregate
results. If there is one generalization possible
from the sub-period analysis for British lamb it
is that the elasticities were lower in the first

Table 4.1: A Sample of the principal price, income and substitution elasticities for meat in the inter-war period

Meat	Price	Income	Substitution	
Lamb				
New Zealand frozen	-1.733	-1.329	British Lamb	-1.303
Australian frozen	-10.886	+15.500	N.Z. Mutton	+0.966
British fresh	-0.889	+0.439	British Mutton	+0.267
Beef				
Argentine chilled	-2.469	+3.348	British Lamb	-4.938
British fresh	-1.531	+0.424	N.Z. Mutton	-0.612
Mutton				
New Zealand frozen	-11.764	+19.376	Aust. Lamb	+0.966
British fresh	-1.152	+1.018	British Lamb	+0.267

period. In other words lamb became more price elastic in the thirties.

A further test and one which is in many ways more rigorous, confirms this tentative result(11). The test is as follows. The years 1920-29, i.e. ten observations, are taken first and the regression equation run. The period was then extended to 1930, the regression re-run, and so on. Thus ten coefficients are obtained. By extending the period by one year in the manner outlined it should be possible to detect which year if any marks a significant change in the coefficient, or alternatively simply to observe the changing pattern in the coefficient. The elasticities are derived from the coefficients in the manner described previously. British and New Zealand lamb, the two principal varieties of this product, were subjected to this method of analysis. The results are interesting in that the price elasticity of British lamb was low to begin with but after 1932 starts to rise and reaches a plateau in the last two years, whereas the New Zealand variety starts off high in the twenties and falls sharply to 1932, thereafter remaining constant and relatively low, throughout the thirties. The sub-period results for mutton were generally good while for beef most of the results were low in statistical significance though where the elasticities were derived they were of the sign and size theory suggests.

To return to the results for the period as a whole an improvement on the first substitutes used in the equations, was to use, not meats of the same variety, but rather those of the same preservation category (fresh, frozen, or chilled). This was an obvious alternative, based on contemporary opinion. For example English lamb would in all probability have been a closer substitute for English beef than was Argentine beef. This was invariably borne out and is reflected in the results.

In general then the results show that the income elasticity for most meats is high - greater than one. The exceptions to this are British beef and lamb. Price elasticities are close to unity for the domestic product but generally much greater for the imported. This is a pattern that might be anticipated; the lower the quality of meat, the greater is the sensitivity to price change, for the greater is the possibility of change to another product. It could be hypothesized that with home produced, fresh, and presumably distinc-

tive varieties of the product there is more stability, less likelihood of major switch away from
the product for a rise in price. Taking this further we might suggest that British beef, mutton
and lamb are the highest quality products. The
only imported items to approach these were New
Zealand lamb and Argentine beef. Though it should
not of course be concluded from these coefficients
that these were the highest quality products of
all, simply that they did compare moderately well
with the home produced meats(12). At the other
end of the scale to these products are Argentine
mutton, which with a positive price coefficient
may be considered an inferior good and Australian
mutton whose elasticity was too high to consider
as seriously belonging to the group. Apart from
these, the poorest quality meats were Australian
and Argentine lamb, and New Zealand mutton.

Much of the above arranging by price elasticities was confirmed by examining the substitution
elasticities that is, that one product at the top
of this ranking was readily substituted by another
and at the bottom of the 'quality' ladder meats
will be readily replaced by one another. (Quality
is used here to suggest a consumer's view, taking
price and some other intangibles into account.
It should not be taken to mean the nutritive value
of the product). For instance the better quality
items, British mutton and British lamb are good
substitutes and at the other end of the scale Australian lamb and New Zealand mutton are close substitutes. These latter results certainly conflict
with the impression left by Stone who shows home
and imported meats of the same variety being readily
substitutable(13). This study shows rather that
fresh meats were close substitutes for one another.
The exceptions are Argentine beef (which was chilled) and New Zealand lamb, the product which took
the freezing process best of all.

Any comparison of the results in this paper
with others is fraught with difficulties, various
investigators having considered different countries
and different periods. Wold and Jureen made estimates for commodities in Sweden both for 1913 and
certain inter-war years. Schultz and Fox made
estimates based on American data for 1922-33 and
1922-41 respectively. Stone made estimates for
the U.K. for 1920-1938 and Philpott and Matheson
produced estimates for the U.K. for 1955-64(14).
Few of these studies used similar classifications
of meat, but even if they had been using strictly

comparable data, differences in income levels between time periods and between countries for the
same period, differences in climate, custom and
so on, all influence income elasticities. For example Wold showed that pork had a significantly
different elasticity in Sweden to what it had in
the United States.

However there are some similarities in the
results, and where patterns are discernible, there
are interesting pointers for further work. Fox,
for instance, points out that as national income
during the inter-war period was fluctuating around
a much lower 'real' level than exists in the years
after 1945, income elasticities should be larger
in the former period(15). Wold came to the same
conclusion, that is that income elasticity for
food and indeed for disaggregated food, presents
a clear tendency to decrease as income grows.
Against this, Wold in separate cross-sectional
studies found similar income elasticity estimates
for the years 1913 and 1933 though he did point
out that 1913 was a prosperous year and 1933 a
depression year.

Stone's results are clearly of most interest
for this study, unfortunately though he simply
made estimates for domestically produced beef and
veal grouped together (income elasticity .34) and
domestically produced mutton and lamb grouped together (income elasticity .70)(16). He then assumed
the imported variety to be identical. Bergstrom
estimated the British demand for New Zealand lamb
in the inter-war period and as in my result, obtained a negative income elasticity, which he explained
in the following way:

> The negative income elasticity of demand for
> lamb is, at first sight, surprising. It should
> be remembered, however, that New Zealand lamb
> is frozen and is likely, therefore, to be
> regarded by United Kingdom consumers as an
> inferior substitute for fresh, home produced
> lamb. Thus it is quite conceivable that an
> increase in the real incomes of United Kingdom
> consumers would, if all prices were held con-
> stant, cause a reduction in the demand for
> New Zealand lamb. In fact of course prices
> would not remain constant, and an increase
> in the United Kingdom real income would, by
> forcing up the price of fresh lamb, cause
> an increase in the demand for New Zealand
> lamb(17).

The statistical confirmation may be satisfying but much else points to the fact that New Zealand lamb was certainly not an inferior good though it may have been a weak substitute for the best fresh variety.

Consumption patterns

The contemporary evidence is of most interest for the light it can cast on consumption patterns. It is perhaps worth stressing that a simple comparison of consumption and income per head over the period is not very helpful for it was precisely the question of separating the effect of income and prices that was tackled in the regression analysis. What such a comparison shows however, is growing income per head but almost static consumption per head of the meats tested.

The problem that arises in an assessment of the contemporary evidence is that of identifying which income groups bought which meats. At first sight this should present no difficulty; we should expect the higher priced and quality meats to move with the higher incomes. The difficulty that arises is that some evidence indicates that this may not always have been the case. Critchell and Raymond remarked of a slightly earlier period, '...but the West-end folk are very large customers for chilled beef of the highest quality and the best grades of New Zealand sheep and lambs'(18). Against this there was the lingering problem of prejudice against the frozen or chilled product and it may be that this 'distorted' expenditure patterns. One possible means of examining the problem is a consideration of cross-sectional income/consumption data for food expenditure patterns for different income groups. Regrettably the evidence is scant. There are some studies of working class budgets but the only survey of the expenditure of middle-class households for this period and in the detail required, does show a steady increase in the total consumption of meat and fish (grouped together) as income increased(19).

A similar pattern emerged from the disaggregated data for individual meats. But there are difficulties for the data are not reduced to a per capita basis and the income groups have not been specified precisely. When the data are reduced to a per capita basis using the figures Massey provides, there are examples of reductions in expenditure per head accompanying increases in income.

Causality cannot be implied for we do not know what the influence of relative price was. No great reliance can therefore be placed on Massey's findings in their present form. But the suggestion implicit from the minor manipulation of the figures is clear: the conventional belief that increasing consumption of meat follows increases in income probably requires qualification when it comes to individual varieties of the product.

It is always difficult to determine the influence of several variables and the most obvious is the problem of relative prices. Where they change substitution may take place either between meats or between meat and other substitutes. One study, of a slightly different kind and covering somewhat different income groups, which contains hints of such behaviour or variations of it (though by no means conclusive evidence) is that of Rowntree(20). Rowntree's study of York in the middle of the 1930s contains interesting information. In a cross-sectional study of different income groups, Rowntree presents four typical budgets showing food expenditure in one week. Extracting the meat consumption from these four typical budgets provides Table 4.2.

Rowntree himself warned against strict comparison of these budgets because of the lack of seasonal uniformity, but it is interesting to note that in this cross-section of income groups there was no clear evidence in support of a positive income/consumption coefficient for the meat under consideration in this paper. In the highest income group there was less meat (as defined for this paper) being bought than there was in the second lowest income group, and in group three there was less bought than in group one. What is evident though is a move to greater variety in meat consumption as income grew; the list of items lengthens as we move across the income scale with some butcher's meat being given up and other categories being introduced. This should not be taken as being in any sense conclusive but it should at least be set against generalizations that are made about this relationship: 'increased purchasing power resulted in greatly increased consumption of...meat, butter, eggs, fruit, vegetables'(21).

One of the most celebrated studies of the 1930s was that of John Boyd Orr(22). Orr stated that, 'consumption of milk, eggs, fruit, vegetables, meat and fish rises with income'(23). And yet there are contradictions in his study. For example

Table 4.2: Meat Consumption in different income groups

Group I (36/- per week) June & September (lb)		Group II (41/8 per week) August (lb)		Group III (72/- per week) May (lb)		Group IV (75/- per week) April/May (lb)	
2.0	roast beef	4.5	roast beef	0.5	stewing steak	2.5	mutton
0.5	liver	1.0	stewing	0.5	best steak	2.0	rabbit
0.5	mince	1.5	sausage	2.0	rabbit	0.5	tripe
0.5	sausage	1.0	liver	1.0	sausage	1.0	pork sausages
0.5	pie	0.5	corned beef	0.25	pork	0.25	corned beef
0.5	bacon	1.5	bacon	0.5	ham	0.75	liver
–		–		1.0	bacon	0.375	ham
–		–		1.0	liver	0.25	brawn
–		–		1.5	hearts	0.25	polony
–		–		–		0.5	bacon
4.5 lb		11.0 lb		8.25 lb		8.375 lb	

Source: B.S. Rowntree, Poverty and Progress (1952) pp. 188-94.

he says 'consumption of milk...does not appear
to have been lower a hundred years ago and in rural
areas was possibly higher'(24). In other words
consumption of milk had fallen or remained static
over a period of greatly rising incomes. Then
again in Orr's cross-sectional studies he does
show meat consumption to be higher in higher income
groups but two points should be made in this connection. The first is that he does not say what
meat is included. The second point is that he
gets the same results for potatoes which of course
is against all the conventional wisdom on potatoes
being the classic example of an inferior good (even
a Giffen good).

Further evidence along the lines above is
provided by Lloyd(25), who showed how consumption
of meat had increased only slightly by 1934-38
compared with 1909-13 and 1924-28. Interestingly
the increase was mainly in bacon and offal, supporting the point made earlier and the suggestion contained in Rowntree's typical budgets. Lloyd posed
the question as to whether this was due to growing
popularity of liver and bacon or to medical recommendation of liver as a cure for anaemia(26).
In summary there is no clear evidence from the
family budget surveys for the inter-war years that
consumption of varieties of butcher's meat rose
or fell with income.

There are of course many remaining difficulties. The problem of taste is undoubtedly complex
but there were other less difficult factors in-
fluencing consumption such as the medical one of
the anaemia campaign which were supported by the
fact that the quality of British beef was said
to be greatly in decline because of the growing
percentage of dairy cattle that was finding its
way into the total. Against what would seem to
be a fairly serious deterioration in the product
has to be set the conservatism of the consumer.
For as Burnett said, 'advertisers would do well
to recognise the force of dietary conservatism
which it seems, expensively mounted campaigns can
influence only marginally'(27). Changes in taste
take place relatively slowly but the dangers of
suggesting that prejudice is stronger than price,
over any long period of time, are great.

In summary, this paper has argued that great
care is necessary in interpreting the evidence
of contemporary studies on the relationship between
consumption of meat and income. Both variables
require careful definition and allowance must be

made for the influence of other variables. The demand analysis of this paper certainly supports much of the contemporary view that the domestic and imported varieties had different markets, and adds some precision to this and other previously accepted positions. However it also demonstrates that there is still much uncertainty over various aspects of demand. Theory was generally vindicated but a remaining difficulty is that a negative income elasticity was obtained for New Zealand lamb (confirming Bergstrom's result) indicating an inferior good and yet this is at variance with some qualitative evidence suggesting that this was one of the very best of the imported preserved meats.

NOTES

1. J.W.F. Rowe, Primary Commodities in International Trade (Cambridge 1965).
2. There is a considerable literature covering supply: Ministry of Agriculture and Fisheries, Agricultural Output and Food Supplies of Great Britain, 1929; R.A. Mackness, 'Beef Supplies in the United Kingdom', Journal of Agricultural Economics, June 1956; R. Duncan, 'The Australian Export Trade with the United Kingdom 1880-1940', Business Archives and History, August 1962; A.W. Flux, 'Our Food Supply Before and After the War', JRSS Vol. XCIII Pt IV 1930; R.J. Hammond, 'British Food Supplies', Econ. Hist. Rev. Vol. XVI No. 1 1946; R.H. Hooker, 'The Meat Supply of the United Kingdom', JRSS 1909; Richard Perren, 'The North American Beef and Cattle Trade with Great Britain, 1870-1914', Econ. Hist. Rev. Vol. XXIV No. 3, 1971.
3. Some work has been done by economists e.g. J.R.H. Shaul, 'The Demand Curve for Beef in Great Britain', Economic Journal, Vol. XIV September 1935; A.R. Bergstrom, 'Supply and Demand for New Zealand's Exports', Econometrica, Vol. 23, July 1955.
4. See for example, J.B. Orr, Food Health and Income (London, 1937); Sir Wm. Crawford, The People's Food (1933); B. Seebohm Rowntree, Poverty and Progress, (1942), discussed later.
5. Board of Trade, Annual Statements of Trade 1920-1940. Supplementary material in International Institute of Agriculture, International Trade in Meat (Rome, 1936) and BPP 1935 Vol. XVII, Cmd 4838. Import of Meat

into the United Kingdom.

6. Ministry of Agriculture and Fisheries, _Agricultural Statistics_, 1922, 1923-25, 1926-28, 1936, 1939, 1939/40-1945/46, Agricultural Output of England and Wales, (1925); Meat, A Review of Production Trade, Consumption and Prices, 1935-1944 (Annually); Marketing of Sheep, Mutton and Lamb, Economic Series No. 29 1931; Marketing of Cattle and Beef, Economic Series No. 20 1929; Trade in Refrigerated Meat (1925).

7. B.R. Mitchell and Phyllis Deane, _Abstract of British Historical Statistics_ (Cambridge, 1970), p. 368; Chapman and Knight, _Wages and Salaries in the United Kingdom_ (Cambridge, 1953), p. 30; J.R.N. Stone, _The Measurement of Consumer Expenditure and Behaviour in the United Kingdom 1920-1938_ (Cambridge, 1954), p. 414.

8. See B.P. Philpott and Mary J. Matheson, _An Analysis of the Retail Demand for Meat in the United Kingdom_ (Lincoln College, New Zealand 1965); G.W. Taylor 'Meat Consumption in Australia', _Economic Record_, March 1963; K. Fox, _Econometric Analysis for Public Policy_ (Iowa, 1958), p. 34.

9. Because of the reversed form of the equation the price elasticity is the reciprocal of the coefficient obtained on quantity and the income elasticity is obtained by using that coefficient and the price coefficient. The signs of the coefficients remain unchanged.

10. F.J. Prevett, 'Consumer Preference; Beef Weights and Prices', _Journal of Ministry of Agriculture_, 1933-34 p. 223.

11. R.L. Brown, J. Durbin, and J.M. Evans, 'Techniques for Testing the Constancy of Regression Relationships over Time', _Journal of the Royal Statistical Society_ Series B 1975.

12. This is confirmed by contemporary opinion, see e.g. Y.F. Rennie, _The Argentine Republic_ (New York, 1945), p. 250, 'At Smithfield the highest priced beef is freshly slaughtered meat from Scotland, which goes to the upper class tables; and next in price and quality i.e. Argentine chilled beef selling for two-thirds as much, and the staple diet of the middle class consumer'; H. Belshaw & others, _Agricultural Organization in New Zealand_ (Wellington, 1936), p. 634.

13. J.R.N. Stone, op. cit.

14. H. Wold and L. Jureen, Demand Analysis: A Study in Econometrics (New York, 1952); H. Schultz, The Theory and Measurement of Demand (Chicago, 1938); K. Fox, Econometric Analysis and Public Policy (Iowa, 1958); J.R.N. Stone, op. cit; B.P. Philpott and Mary J. Matheson, An Analysis of Retail Demand for the Meat in the United Kingdom (Lincoln New Zealand 1965).

15. Fox, op. cit. p. 126.

16. J.R.N. Stone, op. cit.

17. A.R. Bergstrom, 'An Econometric Study of Supply and Demand for New Zealand's Exports,' Econometrica, 1955, pp. 258-271.

18. J.R. Critchell and J. Raymond, A History of the Frozen Meat Trade (1912), p. 279.

19. Phillip Massey, 'The Expenditure of 1,360 British Middle-Class Households in 1938-39', Journal of the Royal Statistical Society 1942 Pt. II, pp. 159-196.

20. B. Seebohm Rowntree, Poverty and Progress (1952) pp. 188-194.

21 John Burnett, Plenty and Want (Harmondsworth 1968), p. 285; Burnett does not say what is included or excluded under 'meat'.

22. John Boyd Orr, Food, Health and Income (1936). This study has been criticized for having an undue proportion of families from the North of England and of families of low earnings.

23. Ibid. p. 49.

24. Ibid, p. 17. In fact Burnett goes further than this when he makes his statement, 'milk was an even better example of the fact that consumption of the most nutritionally desirable foods varied inversely with income', this though would appear to be a mistake on his part, Burnett, Plenty and Want, p. 318.

25. E.M.H. LLoyd, 'Food Supplies and Consumption at Different Income Levels', Journal of the Proceedings of the Agricultural Economics Society, 1936, Vol. IV No. 2. Also quoted in J.C. Drummond and Anne Wilbraham, The Englishman's Food (1964), p. 457.

26. Sir Wm. Crawford in The People's Food (1933) made the same point: 'A greater appreciation of the food value of offals (kidney, liver, etc.) has certainly grown up in recent years, stimulated by the medicinal uses to which they are now put', p. 189.

27. Burnett, op. cit. p. 316.

5. CHANGES IN THE BRITISH BREWING INDUSTRY IN THE TWENTIETH CENTURY

JOHN MARK

Long regarded as a conservative industry using time honoured methods to furnish a traditional product, brewing has in the past quarter century experienced rapid change. Many of its original features, however, remain. Some breweries are integrated backwards into the ownership and management of their own maltings and, with one exception, they control a considerable proportion of the retail outlets for their own products. Typically, they sell through their own tied outlets, through the growing free trade and the even faster growing take home sales from off-licences, supermarkets and shops.

As Table 5.1 shows, at the beginning of the century there were nearly 6,500 breweries with an average output of 5,500 barrels. Although this number had been reduced to 358 in 1960 with an average output of about 71,000 barrels, the majority of the 160 or so firms were of local and regional character. Only in the past fifteen years have the national firms become dominant, to an extent far greater than is indicated by the present number of companies (81) and the number of breweries (142) where brewers for sale licences are currently held by a couple of dozen one man bands. It should be noted that these statistics from the Brewers' Society do not include the rapid growth in the numbers of new small breweries which has been partly inspired by renewed consumer perception of beer. At least 90 small breweries have been established in the past decade or so, mostly involving single houses and the free trade although the estimated 900 outlets do include some significant ties. However, this does not make much difference to the overall fact that the six major companies account for over three-quarters of the total production

Table 5.1: The Changing Structure of the Industry in the United Kingdom

Date	Breweries (Brewers for Sale Licences)	Average output per brewery (1,000 barrels)
1900	6,447	5.5
1910	4,398	8.0
1914	3,746	9.4
1920	2,914	12.0
1930	1,418	17.4
1940	840	29.9
1950	567	45.4
1960	358	70.9
1968	220	136.9
1973	162	214.4
1977	144	271.6
1978	143	281.7
1980	142	293.7

and the 75 regional and local companies the rest. The average output per brewery is around 293,700 barrels, which confirms the dominance of the large companies.

Table 5.2: Concentration Ratios

Percentage Share of the five largest enterprises of the total industry.

	1954	1958	1963	1968	1973	1974	1975
Q Net Output	18	23	50	62	69	60	62
L Employment	19	22	49	61	61	58	56
K Net Capital Expenditure	19	30	52	59	73	64	57

Table 5.2 presents concentration measures computed for brewing and malting from Census of Production data and illustrates the main trends in changes in industrial structure. Using the framework of the neoclassical production function $Q = Q(L, K)$ the first row corresponds to output Q and the second and third rows to labour and capital input respectively. All measures show a

dramatic increase in concentration from 1954 to
1968 with a slight dilution in market dominance
thereafter. The net output measure gives the most
straightforward picture but we would also expect
the net output and net capital expenditure ratios
to be greater than the employment ratio as an indication that the larger firms tend to be more
capital intensive and the smaller firms more labour
intensive. In general this is borne out by the
data with some deviations which may be explained
as follows. The merger boom in the late 1960s
left the major companies with lots of acquired
plant and accompanying labour whence the capital
ratio is lower than the labour ratio for 1968.
But by 1973 much rationalization and investment
had been undertaken hence the return of the order
of the capital and labour ratios to our theoretical
expectations in the most significant manner for
1973 with the capital ratio at 73 per cent and
the labour ratio at 61 per cent. The labour ratio
subsequently behaved as expected but the reduced
capital ratio for 1975 could well be partially
explained by heavier capital investment by the
resurgent regional and local brewers.

Any concentration measure is a summary stat-
istic(1) which conceals important features not
the least of which is the size distribution of
firms and the growth of conglomerate interests.
The measure is an underestimate to the extent that
it does take account of interlocking directorates
(the 'beerage') the significant minority sharehold-
ings in other companies and existing trade agree-
ments. Moreover, and particularly in the 1970s
the straitjacket of the Standard Industrial Classification does not give a full indication of the
market power which flows from diversification into
other fields than brewing and malting. The industry
has sold soft drinks, cider, wine and spirits for
some time but it is the extent to which these and
other activities have grown which is remarkable.
In many respects and notably in the cases of the
major firms, the consumer now faces a leisure industry selling food, accommodation and entertainment, as well as a broad range of alcoholic drinks.

On the other hand, it can be argued that the
simple five firm concentration ratio is an overestimate in that it does not consider competition
from overseas but this is insignificant in the
brewing case since only about 4.5 per cent of beer
consumed is imported. More important, it could
be an overestimate in that it does not give any

weight to any growing intensity of competition of the large firms which could result from any increased equality in their market shares even if the number of firms in the industry has diminished. One cannot draw the same inferences from British data as Ann and Ira Horowitz(2) surmized from their U.S. results which suggested that in spite of the continuing decline in the number of firms in the U.S. brewing industry that relative competition did not suffer as severely because the market shares of surviving firms had become less unequal.

Structural indicators of industrial change provide useful snapshot pictures yet are mere reflections of underlying pressures at work. The main concern is to analyse the importance of four factors: firstly the application of scientific knowledge, secondly the influence of the economies of large scale production, thirdly the marketing environment and the attempts to manipulate tastes and fourthly the impact of government on an industry which has a special fiscal and social significance. But before this is done, it may be useful to see how these factors have reacted with certain financial features.

Takeover bids were often made with an eye on under-valued tied estates yet with the assurance that the overall rate of return on capital could be raised. They placed tempting prospects of gain before equity shareholders in highly geared companies and eased the minds of the owners of family firms hard pressed for the payment of death duties. Whether for reasons of attack or defence, they increased the incentive to adopt new methods of production and to use scientific knowledge to economize in the use of raw materials. These objectives are more likely to be attained by firms large enough to justify the employment of specialists and possessing a capacity which satisfactorily magnifies the small saving per barrel, given that raw material costs have fluctuated between 9 per cent and 15 per cent of the price of a pint of bitter in the period in question. With demand stagnant, or at best slowly rising, markets were primarily extended by the purchase of firms, not so much for their breweries but for their tied outlets and distribution areas. More tied outlets and larger distribution areas intensified the problems of transporting and keeping the beer: these were tackled mainly by infusing draught beer with carbon dioxide at the brewery and serving the beer under pressure ('keg' beer). These keg beers keep longer and can be widely distributed. Furthermore, and most important, the extra outlets and larger areas also required the customer to be persuaded to accept national products, recognizably different from the traditional ales, and this factor increased the role of marketing and advertising. If demand could be increased for a single brew, yielding economies of scale in production, it simultaneously diminished the demand for local brews, whose producers could not afford comparable advertising expenditure. The financial power òf the major companies, especially in marketing, is a crucial feature in recent years.

In the application of scientific knowledge, the search for precision is not at all new but more intense. Peter Mathias(3) has amply described and analysed the increasing exactitude of measurement in the Industrial Revolution period 1700-1830 in an industry which until the last quarter century or so has been regarded as fiercely conservative in its production methods. However it can be argued that Louis Pasteur's influence heralded a new approach which accelerated throughout the twentieth century. His influence was both theoretical (in his Etudes sur la Bière) and practical. In his own words he 'was permitted to go through a large London brewery where the microscopical study of yeast was unknown'. He made 'certain experiments in the presence of the managers' detecting and making diagrams of the micro-organisms found in the yeast'. So impressed were the directors, that eight days later, they purchased a microscope.

Since the publication of Pasteur's Etudes sur la Bière, we can roughly identify three periods. The first, from 1898 to 1920 saw fundamental discoveries in brewing science but little change in well established techniques. The second, from 1920-1930, was characterized by the development of process controls in the brewery based upon technical measures relating to earlier pioneering work, but it is in the third from 1930 onwards that there has been a new positive attitude to applying the fruits of research(4). Led by the formation of the Brewing Research Foundation in 1948 and its establishment at Lyttel Hall in Surrey in 1951, as well as impetus from existing schools of malting and brewing in British Universities, the emphasis has been on 'research' more than 'investigation'. I refer to the much publicized innovations in materials and methods rather than the mere discovery

of the characteristics of traditional ingredients.
In fact, it is no longer sufficient to say
that the raw materials used in the production of
beer are malt, sugar hops and water. Attempts are
continually being made to relate changes in the
mix of ingredients to variations in the taste of
the final product and more will be said in a later
section about efforts by marketing men to determine
what consumer tastes are prior to asking the brewing chemist to find the right formula. This corresponds to the linear programming approach
of selecting that input mix which satisfies requirements at minimum cost. As Table 5.3 clearly shows,
although malting barley is still the most important
constituent, there has been a growth in the use
of unmalted cereals to provide the additional
starches. On the one hand this is not as great
as the rate of change in the U.S. where cereal
adjuncts(5) account for over one third of raw materials but on the other greater than the minimal
usage in West Germany where there is adherence
to their Reinheitsgebot, the purity laws from the
Middle Ages, permitting only barley malt for brewing. But a measure of the degree of substitution
here is that before World War Two, the majority
of the barley crop went to the malster brewer but
the demand for feeding barley today means less
than 10 per cent of the crop is intended for malting
and brewing.

Table 5.3 testifies to the increasing use
of hop powders and hop extracts and the economy
in the use of hops. This flows from the identifica-
tion of the alpha-acids which yield bitterness
and from the isomerising processes. Hop powders
and extracts have clear advantages in their lower
bulk and great uniformity of quality and there
is no disposable problem although spent hops becomes
less available as fertilizer for local farmers.
This innovation is not confined to the large brewers; dissemination of new knowledge is aided by
the spirit of co-operation and interchange traditional in British brewing. Knowledge passes by
example and word of mouth as well as publication.
Also significant as an application of science in
industry is the addition of gibberellic acid which
reduces the length of malting time from nine to
six or seven days. In 1926 a Japanese scientist,
Kurosawa, reported his discovery that an extract
from the fungus Gibberella fugitoroi led to abnormal
growth in rice and other plants. The substance
was crystallized in 1938 and shown to have several

components. The pure extract of one of these components, namely gibberellic acid, was identified chemically in 1950 by Dr. P.W. Brian and a team of biologists from Imperial Chemical Industries which is now one of the world's leading producers of this chemical. In an interesting study on the rate of diffusion, G.F. Ray(6) demonstrates that after the first commercial application in 1959 the leading brewers and malsters began to use the acid to speed up the germination process so that by 1970 this process embraced 80 per cent of U.K. malt production. Medium-sized firms followed to a lesser extent with a four to five year time lag but there was no significant usage by smaller brewers of a process with low capital cost but needing careful specialist supervision.

An understanding of the biochemical properties of the raw materials has had considerable impact. Many strains of yeast have been catalogued, and the culture of a pure form minimizes the danger of beer infection. Advances in process engineering feature routinely in brewing journals and suffice it to say here that up to date equipment from individual vessels to complete computer-controlled breweries yield lower running costs. And although it is true that interest in the application of science is pretty widespread, the larger brewers with greater throughput and greater potential savings benefit most. Therefore it is an appropriate time to turn to the economies of scale in plant although I have not forgotten that brewing is also an art and discuss this later with reference to canons of taste and the resurgence of consumer countervailing power.

Plant economies of scale do militate against the small companies, although all firms have found the necessity of installing new bottling lines and kegging plant financially onerous. Firstly, the fact that the cost of a tank is more closely related to surface area than its capacity, where surface area does not increase proportionately, is obviously applicable to installation costs for a range of vessels. Roughly, if the capacity of a tank is doubled, the cost increases by just over half. With the further bonus that increasing vessel size does not require a proportionate increase in labour force, it is not surprising that with new types of plant, as well as the closure of breweries, net output per head in brewing and malting rose from £2,514 in 1963 to £4,917 in 1970 to £12,295 in 1977. Secondly, the optimal capacity

Table 5.3: <u>Materials used in Beer Production (tonnes)</u>

Year ending 31st March	Malt	Unmalted Corn (a)	Rice, Rice Grits Flaked Rice, Maize Grits, Flaked Maize (a)	Sugar etc. used in brewing
1963	509,062	706	32,734	88,956
1969	577,237	8,906	39,383	108,385
1973	625,498	31,430	20,763	128,067
1978	733,666	41,155	40,789	137,868
1980	758,587	33,341	44,443	131,588

Notes: (a) Before 1973 flaked barley was shown under 'Rice, Rice Grits etc.' but from 1973 flaked barley is included under the 'Unmalted Corn' heading.

(b) Usage of Hop Powder was not significant until the early 1970s and Preparation of Hops (Hop Pellets etc.) became significant from the early 1970s onwards.

Sources: The Brewers' Society, <u>U.K. Statistical Handbook</u> 1975 and 1980 and H.M. Customs and Excise.

Table 5.3. (contd.)

Hops (b)	Hop Powder (b)	Preparation of Hops (b)	Beer Production in Bulk Barrels (millions)
11,510	–	–	27.9
10,739	–	–	32.5
9,325	285	241	35.3
5,942	1,139	759	40.3
5,133	1,156	1,035	41.7

of plant, where several processes and vessels are involved, is the lowest common multiple of the separate capacities of the machines. Whence if the most efficient size for a final process is a large one, it will dictate the number and conceivably the size of other machines. Even if the high capital cost of packaging plant does not precisely set the minimum economic size of the breweries, as in the U.S.A. where an efficient canning line handling 1,200 cans a minute implies the approximate annual output from a single line of one million barrels, nevertheless it cannot be ignored. The fastest canning line in the U.K. is the 1,250 16 oz cans a minute at the £2m Scottish and Newcastle New Fountain brewery in Edinburgh. Thirdly, there can be additional economies of scale in bulk purchase and managerial costs.

Yet the best plant size is that which minimizes combined unit production and distribution costs. Distribution costs fall at first but with the extension of market area rise sharply enough to turn the average total costs curve upwards before production economies are exhausted. The amalgamation and relocation of bottling stores, the centralization of packaging, the palletization of loads and bulk deliveries to larger modern retail outlets are amongst the devices which may check the rate of increase of transport costs but they do not prevent them in the end from rising with the expansion of the distribution area.

The relationship between production and distribution costs helps to explain features of the current structure of the industry. The six national brewers (Division I) and the three large single product specialist brewers (Division II) have national and in some cases international distribution networks. But both the six regional brewers (Division III) and the sixty five small brewers (Division IV) survive where comparatively low distribution costs offset higher production costs. They benefit from compact distribution in well populated areas; Fullers and Youngs of London, Boddington of Manchester, Wolverhampton and Dudley in the Midlands and several firms in the Nottinghamshire area are examples. Or they are protected by their comparative remoteness; Adnams in Southwold, Paine in St. Neots, Elgood in Wisbech and the higher than average survival rate of independents in the West Country are cases in point. Furthermore, there are towns which possess these economic advantages but also are of historic

interest and have civic pride in their own breweries; Harvey of Lewes and Jennings of Cockermouth
for instance. Indeed whole areas where tradition
is important such as the Black Country testify
to the survival of a large regional brewer
in Wolverhampton and Dudley but also other very
small firms like Simpkins of Beverley Hill, Holden
of Dudley, Batham of Brierley Hill and the Netherton
Brewery between Stowbridge and Dudley.
    Despite this, the trend is towards larger-
sized plants. One company which had four breweries
in 1955 and which closed seven of its eleven additional plants since acquired in take-overs had
closed three more by 1976. More recently the Bass
Charrington brewery at Runcorn replaced the brewing
capacity of nine local breweries. The capacities
of three new breweries recently coming into operation range between two and three million barrels
a year. If the minimum efficient size judging
from the most modern plant is thought to be the
2.5 million barrels capacity of the latest brewery,
then with U.K. 1977 production nearly 40.5 million
barrels, an extreme view would be that rationalization should continue until we have no more than
16 breweries. But production economies of scale
myopia should not obscure the lesson of economic
history that, at any point in time in any industry,
there are some firms which are much larger than
the rest. In 1796, the output of Whitbread's new
brewery in Chiswell Street in the City of London
topped 100,000 barrels, which dwarfed many plants
still in operation two hundred years later(7)!
    To turn now to a feature which I believe
dominates all others: the marketing environment.
Without government intervention two contrasting
forces range against one another: on the supply
side the desire of producers to minimize cost by
rigorously pruning the range of products, on the
demand side the desire of fastidious consumers
to maximize satisfaction by the enjoyment of many
different varieties of beer. Since the Monopolies
Commission investigation, the number of brands
has been reduced from some 3,000 in 1967 to the
current 1,500. In fact, the range of basic product
is now even narrower because, by varying the changes
in the post fermentation stages, in the packaging
and in the methods of serving, many additional
products grow from what is essentially one formula
in the brewing process. However, it is prudent
to add that the growth of the lager market is
adding about 50 extra brands to existing numbers.

Advertising has played a crucial role in both the disappearance and the differentiation of products. Intensive publicity for national brands, using all types of advertising from bill boards to television, has had a noticeable impact on the demand for national beers at the expense of regional and local brands. It has been the precursor of take-overs where heavy advertising has contibuted to the rise in demand for the product of a national group with perhaps a trade agreement with and a minority shareholding in a small company. It has been the result of takeovers where acquired breweries have been closed and their separate beers discontinued. The accomplishment of this last process is a matter of commercial judgement and local sensitivity. In some cases, the national product has not immediately replaced the local brews, but a local brew has been replaced by a regional brew which has eventually given way to a national brew. Advertising is both a long-term investment and a current barrier to entry.

From the 1930s to the early 1950s, analysis by type of package showed the falling share of draught and the rising share of bottled beer where national brands in particular had been heavily promoted. Bottled beer which is treated to ease distribution, and storage, and extend shelf life - has an advantage over traditional draught beer which is a living beer fermenting in the cask until it is consumed. Yet the draught/bottled relationship has been reversed from the late 1950s to the present because the industry has found products which enjoy the features of bottled beer without sacrificing the lower transport and handling costs of bulkier containers. Best known is keg beer, treated very much like bottled beer in the brewery, but costing about one-third less to transport as do draught beers which are chilled, filtered and pasteurized in the brewery. Draught dominates in keg, tank and cask, holding nearly 80 per cent share, although the steady decline of bottled is partly attributable in the 1970s to the growth of the take-home market and the increasing use of cans.

Although the compound annual rate of growth of demand from 1960-1980 was about 2.5 per cent the data shows considerable variation when beer consumption is roughly classified by type. The shares of the lower-priced mild (a draught beer which is weaker, slightly sweeter and usually darker than bitter) and brown ale have significantly declined whilst stout and light ale have shrunk to a lesser extent. The Brewers' Society returns for 1959-1972 point to the dramatic growth of 'keg' beer and the gradual increase in bitter where the returns encompass traditional beers, and beers which are chilled, filtered and pasteurized to ease distribution. Thereafter the returns from 1971 to the present lump together all bitters: keg, tank, chilled, filtered, pasteurized and traditional(8). Draught premium bitter, stout and non-premium bitter have had a stable lion's share of the market of between 46 per cent - 49 per cent. And although separate returns are not made to the Brewers' Society most observers think that consumer preference has not only prevented the gradual elimination of traditional beers but that since 1972 there has been a slight increase.

In 1881, Thomas Lamprey, editor of the Brewers' Guardian foresaw the strong possibility that German lager would replace traditional ale in the last twenty years of the century. But if it were not to be then, right now similar prophesies are now being made with more statistical justification. In the last twenty years lager has become the most dynamic product, growing from 2 per cent in 1959 to over 10 per cent in 1973 and claiming over 25 per cent of the market by the end of the 1970s.

It is not too difficult to argue that there may be similar forces at work in the massive devotion of funds to the promotion of lager as there were in the concerted effort to market national keg and premium brewery conditioned beers from the late 1950s onwards. In 1976, TV advertising on lager amounted to £7m which was 36 per cent of the advertising budget for beer for a product with 20 per cent of the market(9). The argument can be modelled by recalling that technical economies of scale fall almost without limit but are more than balanced by rising distribution costs as markets extend. If purchasing power can be gradually transmitted from lower priced to higher priced premium bitter products and now to even costlier lager, whether ordinary or premium, the important transport cost/price ratio will be dragged down.

As well as a conscious marketing drive by the large and specialist firms, the growing popularity of lager may also be partly explained by the appeal to the eye of a clear light liquid which is bright, consistent and cooled; the desire for bland 'clean' products. Lager may also be more acceptable in the growing number of centrally heated pubs and homes and there is a degree of conformism in that all countries outside the British Isles drink predominantly lager. The growing familiarity with lager beer obviously stems from the increase in continental travel. Certainly the substantial investment in lager breweries has to be justified and the product sold and new brewing capacity has had to be added for if ale can be brewed in lager breweries, lager cannot be brewed in ale breweries. Lager breweries require a yeast which settles on the bottom rather than the top of the fermenting vessel. Fermentation time is nearly doubled for this process, and so more capital is tied up. Duty has to be paid before fermentation and there is a time lag before the product can be sold.

The drain on cash reserves in the 1970s whether for new lager breweries or sale under licence is onerous and follows previous heavy expenditure on bottling and canning lines, kegging plant and new style large ale breweries. Advertising is obviously needed once the decision is taken and like 'keg' in the 1960s was aimed at the younger age groups. But it has been increasingly used to broaden the market and to suggest that lager is a seriously manly drink for all weathers and not just the province of teenagers and women and men in hot summers. Premium lagers of greater strength have been launched and brand names such as 'Viking', 'London Lager', 'Norseman', and 'Red Stripe' readily testify to the virility image even in the cases of regional and small brewers who decide, whether readily or not, to follow suit. To be fair, it seems that both producers and consumers expect new products; producers because growth suggests dynamism and success and consumers because new products give an extra sparkle to life. Some sources(10) suggest lager could eventually grow to 75 per cent of the market, yet I favour the S shaped Gompertz learning curve pattern with growth levelling out at around a 30 per cent saturation level despite a sales buoyancy enhanced by the decrease in the lager/draught beer price differential with the rapid upward movement in beer prices.

That draught bitter may well continue to dominate is partly due to consumer countervailing power, checking the inexorable march of the big battalions. A partial explanation of the slight reversal in the concentration of economic power is that many consumers and not only the fanatical, have observed the diminution of taste and aroma and have turned to brewers who use lower proportions of adjuncts and serve beer in the traditional way. Other factors which feature prominently in giving smaller brewers several advantages are as follows. First, they often use durable brewing plant whose capital cost has been written off. Secondly, they have ingeniously redeployed second-hand equipment auctioned off from plants purchased and shut down by the large brewing companies. Thirdly, the locational factors analyzed earlier and understandable local and regional pride and identity means firms do well supplying draught beers at competitive prices, especially to manual workers in urban and rural areas. Fourthly, the consumer movement of the 1960s and early 1970s was inspired by students in Norfolk, deprived of choice by takeovers and rationalization, and journalists and others moving from Manchester to London. This new consumerism accorded well with the desire of people who enjoy good restaurants, tasty cheeses, locally-baked bread and fresh products to seek out traditional brews. If, in the United States, small breweries furnishing high quality, high cost and high priced products can succeed then it is hardly surprising that the quality market is being exploited in the United Kingdom, not only by the regional and local brewers but by the reintroduction of traditional products by the large companies. The latter are often being marketed as new premium products and in some cases the major companies have been compelled to withdraw previously intensively marketed brewery-conditioned beers. Indeed, the experience of the success of smaller rivals during the late seventies and early eighties has prompted changes in the conventional big brewery rationalization and closure familiar in the 1960s. Some large companies have decentralized their marketing regions and revived regional and local trading names. In one case a large company has even set up a small brewery on the premises of one of its public houses. Finally, the smaller brewers enjoy not only the comforting benefit of simplicity but have been producing healthy financial results(11) which have enabled them to expand capacity to satisfy the increased demand. However, the market discipline of fear of take over for the remaining independent companies will never diminish since an attractive way to satisfy a revived traditional market is for the large brewers or even firms outside the industry to purchase a successful local firm.

Now it is time to turn to the role of government which has been substantial ever since Henry VII's statute in 1495 which gave any two justices the power to suppress useless alehouses as part of a policy of 'discouraging indoor games which diverted the people from archery'. The industry has had more than its fair share of government surveillance and intervention. Concern and recommendations have intensified in recent years with ten increases in duty from 1964 to the present, a report from the National Board for Prices and Incomes on cost, prices and profits in the brewing industry in 1966, the Unilever-Allied Monopolies Commission investigation in June 1969, the Monopolies Commission Report on the supply of beer in 1969, the N.E.D.O. Brewery report in 1977, the Price Commission Report in July 1977 on Beer Prices and Margins and the same body's investigation of Allied Breweries UK Brewing and Wholesaling of Beer and Sales in Managed Houses. Of wider social significance there has been the Erroll Report of 1972 and the Clayson Report of 1973.

The revenue yield on alcoholic drinks is vital to the Exchequer reaching as high as 19.8 per cent of all revenue duties in 1970/1971. The beer duty itself is of importance both for the Exchequer and for the structure of the industry. In 1978, beer alone yielded £892.9m slightly more than the £875m yield from whisky. With the VAT revenue which commenced on 1 April 1973, the total yield from Customs and Excise duties plus VAT from beer was some £1,189.7m; which was sufficient to pay for our overseas aid in 1977/78 with some £186.7m over; and which exceeded by some £283.7m the central government expenditure for 1977/78 on agriculture, fisheries, food and forestry(12).

The economic as distinct from the fiscal effects have been five-fold. First, when Gladstone instituted beer duty in 1880 at 31.25p per barrel in place of malt tax, he created the 'Free Mash Tun'. Brewers were henceforth freer to vary inputs according to fluctuations in prices than they had been before. Secondly, the rise in duty, particularly in the two world wars, and the establishment of the progressive nature of duty (the higher the gravity, the higher the duty) were instrumental in the reduction of the strength of beer. Thirdly, it contributed to the drop in consumption and the consequent concentration and mergers when the large number of firms were competing for a declining market, especially in the inter-war years, during

which the general level of prices slowly fell for
a period. Only after the steady climb of consumption in the prosperous sixties and the early seventies did beer production in 1973, for the first
time, surpass the 1900 level. Fourthly, on the
one hand, it may have contributed to concentration
in the years after the Second World War, when consumption was increasing slowly. Any increase in
duty lowers the important transport cost/price
ratio, which is a significant factor in extending
distribution areas. On the other hand, it is possible to argue that the duty's effect has been in
the other direction. The greater the ratio of
duty to price, the smaller is the ratio of raw
materials to price and this lack of incentive to
economize on raw materials may favour the smaller
brewer. This force may have been weakening recently because the incidence of duty, after reaching
a maximum of 37.5 per cent of consumers' expenditure on beer in 1967, has fallen to under 30 per
cent since 1972. Finally, the duty's existence
favours the efficient brewer. The excise authorities permit 6 per cent wastage in their assessment
of the brewer's liability for duty and the actual
wastage in new breweries can be as low as 2 per
cent.
    Nor has the tied house system had a neutral
effect on the structure of the industry. Licensing
by local justices was introduced by Edward VI's
Act in 1552 to deal with 'the intolerable hurts
and troubles to the commonwealth of the realm,
daily growing and increasing'. Controls were dis-
mantled in 1830, but reimposed in 1869 with the
proliferation of ale houses and disorderly
behaviour during the rapid urbanization of the
Victorian era. Throughout late Victorian times
and after the 1904 Act, which was the first to
give the justices power to refuse renewal not only
for misbehaviour but on grounds of social policy,
the scramble for tied outlets with monopoly value
intensified. The 102,000 or so public houses
existing in England and Wales at the beginning
of the century had shrunk to about 66,000 by 1967.
In the same year, brewing companies owned 48 per
cent of all licensed outlets which include full
on licences (mainly pubs), off licences, licensed
restaurants, licensed residential premises, and
so on. Their ownership of 78 per cent of full
on licences and 30 per cent of all off-licences,
certainly eased the problems of demand forecasting
and production planning. But only the Carlisle

State brewery and club brewers formed by the clubs which they supplied entered the industry between 1964 and 1967, and the Monopolies Commission considered that brewery control of retail sales was a serious barrier to entry. However, the ownership of tied outlets did partly protect the smaller brewer and the rate of concentration - so fast in 1969 that, of £754m spent on acquisitions by manufacturing companies, £147m went on drink firms - would have been surely more rapid without the tied house system.

The Erroll Committee was established 'to review the liquor licensing laws of England and Wales'. After a thorough analysis of alcoholic dependence, the slow rise from 1946 in drunkenness, the adverse effect of drink on driving and the connection between alcohol and crime, the Committee nevertheless concluded that most people used alcohol primarily for social purposes and not as a drug. But, although their most publicized recommendations - such as the extension of drinking hours and the lowering of the age limit - have not become law, they have been almost overtaken by commercial and social pressures operating within the existing legal framework. This contrasts with the explicit changes made in Scotland where misuse of alcohol is more serious than in England and Wales, following the Clayson Report. Sunday opening is now allowed and the permitted hours for licensed premises is greatly extended.

In the first place, the number and composition(13) of outlets in England and Wales for the retail trade on the supply of intoxicating liquor has changed and to some degree has diluted the market dominance of the tied estate; a feature stressed by both the Monopolies Commission and the Erroll Committee. Within an overall growth of outlets from 124,017 in 1966 to around 155,000 in 1980, the number of public houses has declined slightly from 66,373 in 1966 to 67,100 in 1980; mostly due to the closure of country inns and redevelopment in inner city areas. Conversely, the justices under the consolidating licensing act of 1964 have seen fit to grant an increased number of residential licences and residential and restaurant licences. The number of registered and licensed clubs rose from 24,190 in 1966 to about 30,000 in 1980 and the number of off-licences grew from 26,590 in 1966 to 33,758 in 1977. The eased availability of beer and alcohol is clearly seen from the substantial involvement of nationwide

supermarket concerns, delicatessens and family
grocers. Brewery ownership of all types of licences
has fallen from 48.3 per cent in 1967 to about
32 per cent in 1980. If the large brewers in Division I have around 75 per cent of all brewery owned
public houses and off licences compared with 65
per cent in 1967, with the growth of the free trade
and other commercial developments overall brewery
ownership of the total number of public houses
and off licences has fallen by more than ten per
centage points from the 65 per cent of 1967. Their
share of off-licences has noticeably declined from
30 per cent in 1967 to just over 11 per cent in
1980 and in a change as dramatic as the growth
of lager sales an unimportant take home market
had grown to 8.5 per cent of all beer sales in
1975. The present figure is about 12 per cent
with 20 per cent currently forecast for the 1980s.

These developments have had a number
of economic consequences, not least the premium
placed on retailing skills. Whilst the eleven
companies studied by the Monopolies Commission
gained a 10 per cent return on capital, compared
with 12 per cent for manufacturing industry as
a whole, the return was much lower on the tied
estate which accounted for 60 per cent of
the capital employed, 33 per cent of the total
cost, but only 10 per cent of the profits. The
Price Commission reiterated this finding in 1977,
reporting a profit margin on capital for brewing
and wholesaling far greater than for retailing,
with figures of 32 per cent and 3 per cent respectively meaning an overall return of some 10 per
cent. Significantly, one of the two large groups
which entered the industry in 1972 (when the £111.2m
for takeovers comprised 9.3 per cent of all U.K.
manufacturing acquisitions in that year) had no
previous experience in brewing. It devised an
accounting system which separated production from
retailing and rapidly became one of the most profitable companies. With the exception of Carlisle
State Brewery, a thriving business broken up amongst
existing brewers, the firms which expanded and
entered the industry by acquisition have been outsiders from the hotel, food, tobacco and leisure
sectors. This has intensified the thrust to manage
a greater proportion of the tied estate as well
as other activities to extend the market which
include the acquisition and improvement of hotels,
supplying clubs tied by loan and making supply
contracts with supermarket chains. The latter is

the most competitive section of the business where
lager has the greatest share yet where margins
are the lowest.

In conclusion, the public house still
flourishes but no longer has a virtual monopoly
over the consumption of alcohol. National brewers,
as increasingly conglomerate producers and retailers
have penetrated their products into the home via
the buoyant take home market, not without some
disquieting signs of a connection between
the greater availability of drink and the growth
of alcoholic dependence and convictions for drunkenness. The industry is roughly divided into two
sectors where the first sector of dominant firms,
in most cases more so than the rest, have increased
their production and marketing of other beverages
and leisure products:- wine and spirits, cider
and perry, soft drinks, food interests and entertainment. Their rate of return on capital is a
secure 9 per cent - 13 per cent which is 4 per
cent below manufacturing industry as a whole. They
share the characteristic of diversified leading
conglomerates and giants for the British economy
as a whole that their profits are more secure but
below average(14). Change is symbolized in the
switch in emphasis of many English public houses
from the dart playing, beer drinking atmosphere
to food and musical entertainment. Yet tradition
still flourishes and is reviving somewhat in the
second and smaller sector of the brewing industry.
Proud local and regional brewers, more specialist
and profitable than the others, flourish in an
age where the number of educated and discriminating
consumers are growing.

Notes

1. P.F. Hart, M.A. Utton and G. Walshe, Mergers
    and Concentration in British Industry (Cam-
    bridge, 1973), pp. 18-21.
2. A. and I. Horowitz, 'Entropy, Markov processes
    and competition in the brewing industry',
    Journal of Industrial Economics 16 (1968),
    pp. 196-211.
3. P. Mathias, The Brewing Industry in England
    1700-1830 (Cambridge, 1959).
4. See J.S. Hough, D.E. Briggs and R. Stevens,
    Malting and Brewing Science (1971).
5. For a definition of adjuncts see Ministry
    of Agriculture, Fisheries and Food, Food
    Standards Committee Report on Beer (1977).

6.   L. Nabsett and G.F. Ray (eds.), The Diffusion
      of New Industrial Processes: an International
      study (Cambridge, 1974).
7.   Mathias, op.cit.
8.   It is important to note the following
      conceptual distinctions. The term 'brewery-
      conditioned draught beer' covers all chilled,
      filtered and pasteurized beers including keg
      and tank. The term 'cask-conditioned draught
      beer' means traditional beers which mature
      naturally.
9.   J.Q. Walker, 'The Lager Market', Brewers'
      Guardian (1978).
10.   D. Churchill, 'Changing demands in beer con-
      sumption', Financial Times, 23 March 1979.
11.   Besides numerous stockbrokers' reports, the
      Price Commission (1977) showed that net profit-
      ability per wholesale pint was inversely
      related to size.
12.   Expenditure Plans 1979-80 to 1982-83, Cmnd.
      7439 (1979), pp. 34-5 and 42-3.
13.   Many of the statistics which follow are
      derived from the Brewers' Society, U.K. Stat-
      istical Handbook (1980).
14.   See G. Meeks, 'Giant Companies in the U.K.
      1948-1969', Economic Journal, December 1975;
      G. Meeks, Disappointing Marriage: A Study
      of the Gains from Merger (1979).

6. THE PRODUCTION AND MARKETING OF FRUIT AND VEGETABLES, 1850-1950

PETER ATKINS

Historians of the British diet have found it difficult to assess the contribution played in the past by fruit and vegetables. There is a lack of reliable data on amounts consumed before the early part of the twentieth century, and our knowledge of former cooking practices and their effect upon the nutritional value of consumption is scanty or based upon guesswork. Even the supply system of horticultural products has not received the attention from economic historians that it deserves as one of the most rapidly growing sectors of agriculture during the period 1850 to 1950. The aim of this paper is to describe both the changing location of production and marketing system, and thereby to throw light upon some of the factors which influenced the evolution of demand for fruit and vegetables.

Horticulture around London

An important and lasting contribution to the study of spatial patterns in the location of agricultural production was made in 1826 by J.H. von Thünen in his book Der Isolierte Staat in Beziehung auf Landwirtschaft und Nationalokonomie. This work centred on an analysis of the effect upon its land-use of a farm's distance from market and the cost of transporting its produce to the consumer. Von Thünen formulated a spatial model in which the identified concentric belts of land-use deployed around a focal point of demand, and showed directly and indirectly that the relative location of enterprise types depended among other things upon the perishability of their product, its suitability for transport, its bulk to value ratio, and the potential for a further intensification of produc-

102

tion(1). He predicted that market gardening would
be found close to urban markets:

> Delicate horticultural products such as cauli-
> flower, strawberries, lettuce, etc., would
> not survive long journeys by wagon. They
> can moreover, be sold only in small quantities,
> while still fresh ... Gardens will therefore
> occupy the land immediately around the
> town(2).

The crude economic and behavioural simpli-
fications made in this model are such that one
would not expect Von Thünen's rings to be mirrored
in the land-use maps of the real world. His work
does, however, provide a useful first approximation
of patterns around the London of his time, given
the inevitable variations in soil fertility and
ease of transportation which disturbed the ideal
pattern(3). One can readily identify competition
for land near the city by brick-making, dairying
and market-gardening, with specialization in
successively more distant parishes upon hay production and intensive arable cultivation. The inner-
most ring was not, however, exclusively devoted
to one form of land-use, but rather divided in
a sectoral fashion into an area to the north and
north west of the city where dairying predominated
on pastures growing in clay soils, and an elongated
zone of market gardens and nurseries occupying
the terrace-gravels and brickearths within two
miles either side of the river Thames(4). Here
the soils were easier to work, better drained,
and 'warmer' than the London Clay of surrounding
districts. Access to the river was an important
factor: fruit and vegetables were exported and
the town stable and cowshed manure, so vital for
conserving the fertility of the garden grounds,
was imported more cheaply than would have been
possible by road.

Even in the mid-nineteenth century the concentration of British market gardening in the immediate environs of London was remarkable. One writer
estimated that there were over 12,000 acres devoted
to the production of culinary vegetables (as distinct from vegetables produced as feed for the 20,000
cows housed in London) and 5,000 acres of tree
and bush fruit close to London(5). Charles Whitehead called the area within a carting distance
of fifteen miles the 'charmed circle'(6). Horticulture was attracted here for a number of reasons.

First, the perishability of the produce was a vital factor: growers were reluctant until late in the nineteenth century to take the risk of sending their fruit and vegetables from further afield because of the slowness of transport and the primitive accommodation offered by the railways. An exception to this rule was the large-scale trade by road which developed in the hardy fruits, especially apples, between Kent and London after the Napoleonic wars. Secondly, the cost of transporting manure from London rose steeply over a short distance. This was an important consideration in the cost structure of market gardening because anything up to one hundred tons per acre were applied for some crops(7). A third factor was the readily available pool of casual labour in the city. This not only facilitated the gathering of crops, but also made possible the very intensive form of spade cultivation characteristic of the market gardens around London.

The rewards could be substantial from this type of horticulture, especially where growers indulged in the speculative production of delicate luxuries like asparagus. On the other hand the costs were also considerable, because market gardening was both capital - and labour-intensive. Rents were high as a result of the competition for land around London with users of land such as cowkeepers, brickmakers, and of course builders. The majority of growers who were not owner-occupiers were unable to buy security at any price, however, because the most common form of tenurial agreement contained a 'resumption clause' by means of which the landlord was entitled to resume possession at short notice(8). The development of sites for housing, industry or other urban uses was therefore a constant threat(9). The response to these pressures market gardeners developed intensive methods of cultivation, such as the forcing of valuable vegetables and fruit with the aid of glasshouses, or grew crops which would give a rapid return on investment. In this way most derived a good income and were able to pay their rent. Their success is shown by the ability of horticulture to survive in the interstices of London's expanding urban area in the late nineteenth and early twentieth centuries.

London's market-orientated fruit and vegetable belt remained more or less intact until the final third of the nineteenth century. It is interesting to note that within this belt there was a greater degree of spatial complexity in the land-use pattern than predicted by von Thünen. C. Whitehead noted, for instance, that around the city there was an inner circle of spade cultivation where the most delicate vegetables requiring the most attention were grown, such as asparagus, sea-kale, French beans, celery, radishes, lettuces, and mustard and cress(10). Beyond this was a zone of plough cultivation producing the more bulky and less perishable crops such as peas, beans, onions, brussels sprouts, broccoli and cauliflowers. The outermost ring was devoted to the less valuable vegetables, grown in ordinary rotations, including cabbage, potatoes, turnips, and carrots. Soft fruit was common in the outer zones, but tree fruit was less likely to be found near the city because of the long time lag between the planting and maturation of fruit trees.

In addition to this gradation of crops with distance from market, a further element of complexity was the result of specialism by district, in response to soil type, microclimate, or simply entrepreneurship. Mortlake was renowned for its asparagus, Battersea for cabbage and cauliflowers, Deptford for onions, Mitcham for herbs, Charlton for pears, Dagenham for potatoes, and sea-kale was grown on the Jamaica Level(11).

In the final third of the nineteenth century this necklace of gardens around the metropolis was broken(12). A number of factors were responsible: the rising cost of labour which encouraged a substitution of the plough for the spade and therefore reduced the competitive advantage of the intensive small-scale growers; renewed urban pressure which forced up the rent of suitable land, especially during upswings of the building cycle; the improved facilities for the transport of perishable produce provided by the railway companies, which made the rural producer competitive in London's markets for the first time(13); and the decline in the early twentieth century of the town as a source of cheap manure. By 1900 the modified von Thünen pattern of sectors and more or less concentric land-use zones had dissolved, although substantial pockets of fruit and vegetable cultivation continued to thrive in west Middlesex, the Lea Valley, and north-west Kent(14).

Expansion away from London

The last two or three decades of the nine-

teenth century saw a rapid and unprecedented expansion of market gardening in provincial England(15).
This was encouraged by the push factor of a general
depression in agriculture from the mid-1870s, which
forced farmers into those sectors such as dairying
and horticulture which still offered some profit.
The pull factor of concentrated and accelerated
demand in urban areas was another important consideration.

The option of producing fruit and vegetables
for human consumption was not open to all farmers.
Areas distant from market, with cold, heavy clay
soils, or with a short growing season were unlikely
to have succeeded in what became a very competitive
industry. Large tracts of the country, however,
were basically suitable for horticulture, and the
pattern of localization in the period 1850 to 1920
therefore requires some explanation.

Physical factors Some areas were particularly favourable for market gardening or fruit cultivation
by virtue of their soil fertility. This was true
for instance of north Kent between Rainham and
Faversham where deep loams and brickearths were
well suited to the cherry, perhaps the most demanding of all tree fruits grown in Britain. Other
horticultural crops are not as sensitive to the
chemical properties of the soil, especially if
the grower (and consumer) is satisfied with a less
than top quality product, and for them any 'tractable' soil is adequate. R.R.W. Folley defines
a tractable soil as one which is easy to work,
quick in drying, not subject to panning in its
structure, and capable of improvement(16). Bedfordshire is a good example of a market gardening region
which grew in the late-nineteenth century in spite
of, rather than because of the qualities of its
soil. The light hungry soils of the Lower Greensand
were easily worked, but lacked organic content,
and their fertility was in effect artificially
created by the addition of stable manure imported
by railway from London.

Climatic variation is a great deal more difficult to control, and this factor is the most significant in determining changes in yield from season
to season. Freedom from frost in spring is important for fruit and for certain sensitive vegetables
like cauliflower, but certain frost-free sites
like sea coasts may be exposed to strong winds
and therefore be equally unsuitable, or like hill-
slopes their degree of elevation may reduce the

length of the growing season below a desirable
threshold. Light intensity is another key variable,
but a high light intensity may be a mixed blessing,
because in our climate long periods of sunshine
are usually also periods of dry weather(17). Lack
of soil moisture, causing checks in growth especially in shallow rooting crops, was a serious problem
for farmers in the period before spray irrigation
became possible with the technical advances of
the mid-twentieth century.

At a meso-scale, climate may account for the
fact that British orchards and soft fruit have
a more southerly centre of gravity than is true
of the location pattern of vegetables, because
warm weather in spring and summer has a greater
effect upon the yield of fruit trees and bushes(18).
It may even be cited as evidence accounting for
local pockets of horticulture, such as the glasshouse industry on the south coast, especially around
Worthing where the light intensity is at a maximum,
or the areas of early production such as Cornwall
where the winters and springs are relatively mild
and frost-free. But climatic variations are by
no means a sufficient explanation of the spatial
pattern of production, especially in the period
after the 1890s when an increasing proportion of
output has come from the controlled environment
of glasshouses spread through the country.

One suspects that these physical factors,
other than in a few isolated cases, were no more
than 'permissive' influences upon the location
of horticultural districts. If the conditions
of climate and soil were right, or even slightly
sub-optimal, as they were over large areas of the
country, then ceteris paribus fruit and vegetable
production was feasible. This was especially true
in the middle of the nineteenth century when the
relative advantages of particular areas were untried
and farmers therefore did not know if they would
be able to compete in the market successfully.
By the 1930s, however, the uncertainty had been
reduced and crops were increasingly grown in those
localities which were able to meet their individual
requirements. Several notable discoveries had
been made of areas with great potential: for instance in the Isle of Ely celery was grown by then
on the black fens around Littleport, and soft fruit
at Wisbech(19).

Other factors One all-pervading necessary condition
of production in the provinces, certainly in the

period 1880 to 1920, was proximity to a railway station. This was important for the prompt and rapid export of produce, even though there were constant complaints about the costly and often inconvenient nature of the service provided. The railway was also used for the importation of town manure until this source was cut off by the revolution in road transport in the early twentieth century. Once again Evesham was fortunate in its access to railway facilities. It had fourteen stations within a radius of five miles, and was well connected with the lucrative markets of the Midlands, South Wales, and the northern industrial cities, many of which had poorly developed local supplies of fruit and vegetables.

The exploratory process of trying new crops in areas which had no previous experience of intensive cultivation was responsible for some unusual locational developments, especially in the nineteenth century. An example of this was the rhubarb industry of the West Riding, which developed in the 1820s in the country between Leeds and Wakefield. It grew from the initiative of a few farmers for whom forcing rhubarb was a sideline to their main enterprise, and by 1950 about 5,000 acres were devoted to this one crop. The nature of the cultivation was entirely artificial, because the rhubarb was forced in sheds on a free draining and acidic soil created by the addition of substantial quantities of ashes and soot(20).

Once a local specialism of this sort has become established it may persist even if the initial locational advantages are gone. Growers will be reluctant to write off the capital they have tied up plant, or the local skill in cultivation, harvesting and marketing which is acquired. A good quality product will bring the region a reputation and possibly favourable connections in the city markets where quality and reliability are at a premium. These accumulated advantages may even be sufficient to give an advantage over competitors with lower costs who may find it difficult to become established in the face of an existing monopoly. Examples of specialized areas that have survived for decades in this way include the Lea Valley (glasshouse tomatoes and cucumbers) and Bedfordshire (brussels sprouts)(21), while fruit growing has persisted for centuries in Kent.

Another factor worthy of consideration is the nature of the entrepreneur responsible for the diffusion of fruit and vegetable growing in provincial Britain. In the late nineteenth and early twentieth centuries he was typically a small-holder, and often a former farm labourer, who wished to make the maximum use of the limited resources of land and capital at his disposal. This he did by the substitution of a heavy input of labour, often including that of his own family, but rarely with any hired help. Such an enterprise may have started as a part-time use of the cottage garden and subsequently grown to a fully fledged market garden. The available evidence suggests that this process was common in several districts in the late nineteenth century, notably in the Vale of Evesham (asparagus), south Hampshire (strawberries), and Wisbech (soft fruit), and in other areas where the crop did not require a heavy initial outlay of capital. The provision of additional smallhold-ings by County Councils in the twentieth century was the result of the Small Holdings and Allotments Acts after 1892, especially that passed in 1908.

Emergence of specialized districts

By the outbreak of the First World War several horticultural districts had emerged to challenge the traditional supremacy of the London region and Kent. The Vale of Evesham in Worcestershire was the most important single concentration of market gardening outside the south-east, specializ-ing in plums and asparagus(22), but other substan-tial contributions were made by Bedfordshire (onions, and brussels sprouts)(23), Cornwall (broccoli)(24), the Channel Islands (new potatoes, and tomatoes)(25), south Hampshire (strawberries) (26), and Wisbech and Cambridgeshire(fruit)(27), with smaller pockets scattered throughout the coun-try(28). Complementary to these specialist dist-ricts there developed in the first half of the present century a large scale horticultural industry based upon the use of glasshouses, for instance around Worthing and in the Lea Valley. This required substantial capital investment, but made possible the cultivation of fruits and vegetables such as grapes, tomatoes and cucumbers, whose yields were uncertain when grown in the open air(29). After the First World War a new pattern of horticultural production began to evolve. Veg-etables which hitherto had been the exclusive con-cern of the market gardener were increasingly grown in arable rotations by farmers whose main commit-ments were not in intensive cropping. The eastern counties, especially Norfolk, Suffolk and parts of Lincolnshire, along with the Lancashire moss-lands, were the main beneficiaries of this trend. A major contributory cause was the increasing use of the motor lorry, which for the first time freed the grower from the constraint of needing to be close to a market or a railway station. Other factors were the innovation of mechanical planting, cultivating and harvesting aids which reduced the necessary labour input, and the spread in the 1930s of canning, bottling and other processing plant to these promising new producing areas. This latter development encouraged a greater degree of local-ization in the way that jam-making factories had for soft fruit in the 1880s, and quick-freezing plant was to do for peas and beans in the 1950s(30).

It was the cheaper and bulky vegetables which increasingly came to be produced extensively by arable farmers. They tended to specialize in one or two crops and were able to compete successfully with the market gardener whose unit costs were greater. In consequence the specialist horticul-tural districts were forced to concentrate on grow-ing the more valuable and perishable crops such as lettuce, salad onions, radishes, celery, rhubarb, leeks and runner beans(31). Ironically the growers of the London region had suffered a similarly pain-ful transition in the 1870s and 1880s when competi-tion from produce imported by rail had become severe.

By the mid-twentieth century a number of high-ly-localized specialisms had emerged as a result of the search for suitable locations, the competi-tion between arable and market gardening districts, and the development of new marketing structures. For instance, approximately three-quarters of the celery grown in England and Wales came from within twenty miles of Littleport in the Isle of Ely; two-thirds of the carrot supply originated in the Isle of Ely and adjacent parts of Cambridgeshire, Huntingdonshire, west Norfolk and Suffolk; two-thirds of the country's home-grown cauliflowers were from small coastal pockets of land in Lincoln-shire, Kent and Cornwall; and over half of our brussels sprouts come from farms within a fifteen mile radius of Biggleswade.

In fruit-growing there was a similar although less significant trend of extensive cultivation in soft fruits such as blackcurrants. Moreover a shift eastwards in the centre of gravity of orch-ards and soft fruit growing has been discernible in the twentieth century. This has been due in the case of apples and pears to the increased popularity amongst growers for high quality dessert fruits rather than the coarser vintage fruits which were concentrated in the orchards of farmers in West Country counties such as Devon, Somerset and Hereford.

Marketing

The marketing of fruit and vegetables was a relatively simple operation so long as market gardening was concentrated in the immediate vicinity of the large urban centres. In 1850 about 80 per cent of London's supply came from a short distance by road and water(32), and even in the 1880s a fair proportion of sales in Covent Garden were by the growers themselves(33). But as the suburban grower was pushed further from the centre of the city by the spread of the built-up areas, and as provincial horticulture began to compete, so there developed the need for one or more intermediaries between producer and consumer. This need was felt first in London, where as early as 1839 there were 80 specialized commission salesmen in Covent Garden alone(34).

By 1900 a sophisticated trade had developed, centred mainly on London, and specialized not only in the type of produce sold, but also in the sorts of transaction. It is the purpose of the following paragraphs to outline the great variety of marketing channels which developed in the period 1850-1950(35).

Assembly

Many provincial growers, whether they sold their output to London or some other city, dealt directly with the wholesale market. This was likely where it was practicable to deliver by road in the grower's own transport, or where there were well-established links with individual wholesale traders. Small-scale producers in districts remote from the consuming centres, however, found it increasingly convenient in the twentieth century to dispose of their goods locally. As the scale of the industry grew, so it became feasible for buyers to tour market gardens and orchards contracting for produce sufficient to meet the predicted demand of urban consumers. Many merchant buyers were able to operate on their own account and, if their capital allowed, offered services such as the provision of empty packages and skilled harvesting gangs. On occasion they even bought a growing crop. Buyers who lived and worked in one district frequently acted as agents for town-based wholesalers and were required to supply regular and pre-specified quantities. In this way they were able to provide a certain link between the producer and his market above and beyond their nominal function of bulking. In some areas, Bedfordshire in particular, a small number of market gardeners extended their operations into the wholesale of the vegetable output of their smallholders colleagues(36). This was a development of the 1930s when the motor lorry gave a greater degree of flexibility to collection rounds.

Another form of rural assembly available from the early twentieth century was the local auction market, whether privately owned or operated by a producers' co-operative. By 1927 there were 17 in the west Midlands alone, handling between a quarter and a third of all the fruit and vegetables sold in Worcestershire and adjacent counties(37). This area was also in the forefront of the development of horticultural co-operative societies, of which twenty were affiliated to the Agricultural Organization Society by 1911(38). These organizations provided valuable assistance to their members in the bulk purchase of necessary inputs, but many were also geared to the collection and marketing of produce. Their mixed success, however, was a function of the high basic costs inevitably involved in a large number of small transactions, and the difficulty of enforcing regulated marketing processes, such as uniform packing and grading, upon a large and disparate membership of smallholders. By the 1950s several of these co-operative societies had become large and efficient wholesale businesses selling in the traditional markets or direct to supermarket chains(39).

Wholesale distribution

A fundamental difficulty in describing the wholesale trade in fruit and vegetables is that a large proportion of wholesale traders perform more than one function. The classification adopted here should not, therefore, be regarded as more than a convenient way of describing the broad structural outlines of the trade.

Commission salesmen, who operated in all the whole-

sale fruit and vegetable markets from a very early
date, were a vital link in the marketing chain.
They sold produce, especially for the growers who
had no opportunity to visit the market themselves,
on a commission which varied between 5 and 10 per
cent, depending on whether they provided empty
packages. These salesmen, located as they were
in the consuming centres, were in a position to
provide several useful services to the grower.
First, they had regular and extensive contacts
with wholesale merchants and retailers in the area
served by the market. They were thus well informed
about market conditions and could usually arrange
a quick and advantageous sale. This role was enhanced in some cases by salesmen specializing in
particular commodities such as Evesham asparagus,
or Eastern Counties celery, and their skill was
therefore highly refined. Secondly, they were
able to deal with large quantities of produce,
and usually had warehouse accommodation in or near
the market, where stocks could be held for a steady
rate of disposal(40).
        The basic role of the commission salesmen
was that of urban-based assembly. He often drew
his supplies from a large number of growers, and
it seems that the majority of the long-distance
trade was carried on in this way. In the 1950s
68 per cent of Bedfordshire produce passed through
the hands of commission agents, a proportion which
in West Cornwall was 71 per cent, in the Wisbech
area 70 per cent, and in the Lea Valley 88 per
cent(41).

Wholesale merchants operated in more markets than
commission salesmen. Their function was concerned
less with the assembly of goods than with the sub-
division and dispersal of the precise quantities
required by retailers, hotels, restaurants and
other purchasers of fruit and vegetables(42). In
order to meet the regular and fluctuating demands
of their customers, wholesalers needed widespread
contacts, and bought from brokers, commission salesmen, and the various forms of rural assemblers
described above. Their trade involved considerable
risks in view of the often dramatic fluctuations
of supply and demand, and the investment of capital
was therefore necessary to enable the holding of
stocks. A wholesaler's day to day overheads were
also substantial because of the administrative
and clerical costs of dispersing of produce in

relatively small quantities to a large number of customers.

Commission buyers were mostly based either at Covent Garden or the port auctions. They acted as agents for provincial wholesalers who were unable to attend these markets, and relied for a living upon their specialized knowledge of where and when to buy most cheaply on behalf of their principal. The import trade was largely in the hands of brokers, whose function was to receive the produce and dispose of it either by auction or private treaty at the port of entry, at Covent Garden, or the London Fruit Exchange in Spitalfields. They acted on behalf of overseas shippers at a 5 per cent commission, or imported on their own behalf. The international connections of the trade were such that in 1926 it was reported that brokers were competing with each other for the produce of foreign growers by making advances to them for packing and transport, and by employing agents in the producing areas to protect their own interests(43).

Urban wholesale markets

The fruit and vegetable markets of London lost their importance as centres of retail distribution early in the nineteenth century. By 1850, at the beginning of our period, the wholesale trade dominated the major markets of Covent Garden, the Borough and Spitalfields, and later spread to local markets such as Greenwich and Brentford, and to markets set up on railway premises at Kings Cross (L.N.W.R., 1865), Stratford (G.E.R., 1879) and Somers Town (M.R., 1892)(44).

In the main these markets were complementary in function. Their relative location, for instance, arranged around the central city core ensured a degree of local spatial monopoly: Covent Garden served inner west London, the Borough satisfied the needs of south London, and Spitalfields was orientated towards the East End. Even the type of produce sold was not identical in each market, as shown in 1851 by Mayhew (Table 6.1). The Borough and Spitalfields specialized in the heavy, cheaper vegetables suitable for the poor districts in which they were situated. Farringdon and Portman were small markets which had developed an expertise in a limited range of fruit and vegetables such as broccoli, watercress, cucumber and nuts. Covent

Garden was the major centre of distribution for
24 out of the 36 times listed by Mayhew.
Covent Garden market had been chartered in
1670, and from its earliest days had been the most
successful of London's horticultural markets(45).
In 1850 it was responsible for about 45 per cent
of London's wholesale fruit and vegetable turnover,
more than double that of its nearest rival Spitalfields. In the period 1850 - 1950 Covent Garden
developed four main types of trade, all but the
first of which were also to be found to some extent
in London's other markets.

1. Scarce and exotic fruits and vegetables, often
   unobtainable in other markets. Such was the
   renown of Covent Garden for high-quality luxury
   produce that supplies were re-consigned to
   markets in provincial cities.
2. Produce of the market gardens around London:
   mainly for consumption in London itself.
3. The main crop from provincial market gardening
   and farming districts.
4. Imported produce, especially fruit.

   In the second half of the nineteenth century
Covent Garden attained a national reputation amongst
growers and salesmen which was enhanced by the
centrality of London in the railway network and
the rapid dissemination of information about prices
and available supplies made possible by the telegraph and later the telephone.
   Marketing developments in provincial cities
were years or even decades behind those of London.
This was a function not only of retarded technical
innovations of organization, but also of the limited
possibilities available for local entrepreneurs
in areas where concentrations of demand were small.
In consequence, growers saw the London market as
their main hope of a substantial and sustained
demand, and the inevitable result was an over-
concentration of produce in already overcrowded
markets like Covent Garden, causing periodic gluts
in London when at the same time markets in other
cities were poorly supplied.
   The salesmen based in London's markets did
not discourage this 'market-chasing', as it was
called. They benefited in fact, because by 1900
an efficient re-distribution trade had developed
in which produce surplus to the requirements of
the capital's needs was sent back to the provinces.
Gradually London became the principal node

Table 6.1: The Quantities of Home Grown Fruit and Vegetables
sold in London's Wholesale Markets, 1851

(Quantities in tons, unless otherwise stated)

Fruit	Covent Garden	Borough
Apples	9,000	625
Pears	5,750	250
Cherries	482	241
Plums*	2,325	388
Gages*	50	8
Damsons*	495	79
Bullace+	45	41
Gooseberries	3,500	655
Red Currants*	438	94
Black Currants	281	75
White Currants	24	19
Strawberries	285	147
Raspberries	10	2
Mulberries	8	26
Hazel Nuts	1	-
Filberts	99	32
Total	22,792	2,681

Vegetables		
Potatoes	72,000	21,600
Cabbages	30,000	17,143
Broccoli and Cauliflowers	4,018	8,438
Turnips	25,179	6,429
Turnip Tops	670	1,116
Carrots	5,357	701
Peas	2,411	446
Beans	893	179
French Beans	938	64
Veg. Marrows	145	43
Asparagus	161	48
Celery	335	107
Rhubarb	161	1,071
Lettuces	328	482
Radishes	46	289
Onions	12,500	9,950
Spring Onions	16	5
Cucumbers	1	5
Herbs	48	64
Watercress (thou.bunches)	1,578	180
Total (excl. watercress)	155,205	68,181

Notes: * not all home grown + wild plums
Sources H. Mayhew, London Labour and the London Poor vol.I
(1851) 80-1; B. Poole, Statistics of British Commerce
(1852) 167 & 309.

Table 6.1: (Contd.)

Spitalfields	Farringdon	Portman	Total
6,250	875	400	17,150
2,075	500	250	8,825
80	64	60	928
1,125	75	500	4,413
38	25	13	133
113	225	30	941
10	14	14	123
2,288	300	175	6,918
469	38	56	1,094
281	38	25	700
94	19	13	168
177	7	66	682
1	2	1	16
3	8	10	54
–	2	–	4
19	64	17	231
13,022	2,254	1,629	42,379
28,800	10,800	5,400	138,600
10,714	7,500	14,707	80,064
6,429	11,875	1,219	31,978
6,429	4,688	1,002	43,725
1,339	558	446	4,129
1,071	670	244	8,043
893	125	36	3,911
89	21	9	1,191
80	335	64	1,481
48	6	24	266
14	19	19	262
134	67	134	777
643	54	107	2,036
926	58	212	2,006
241	121	193	890
10,000	240	4,550	37,240
10	10	6	47
11	5	17	39
63	52	26	254
180	12,960	60	14,958
67,934	37,203	28,416	356,939

of articulation in the national distributive network, although this was a development not necessarily in the interests of efficiency for two reasons.
First, it was not until the twentieth century that
cross-country consignments were made on a large
scale. Most goods that were not sold in local
markets before this were sent to London, adding
to the eventual cost to the consumer. Secondly,
some provincial wholesalers found it easier to
import produce from London than to persuade local
farmers to grow fruit and vegetables. In 1880 J.Page
noted that vegetables that could well have been
grown near Manchester, such as rhubarb, lettuce,
runner beans, and brussels sprouts, were all imported via London(46). In the subsequent two decades,
however, it is interesting to note that Manchester,
in common with several other British cities, did
develop its own autonomous links with market gardens
in other parts of the country, and local growers
were encouraged to expand their output to satisfy
the substantial demand of the urban-industrial
belt of southern Lancashire. Only the choice and
early produce was sent from London in 1897(47).

Retail distribution

The perishability of most fruit and vegetables
and the poorly developed system of distribution
meant that retail sales were highly centralized
in most British cities in 1850. Producer-retailers
held sway in the trade outside London until late
in the nineteenth century when middlemen developed
a recognizably separate function for the first
time and retail shops challenged the monopoly of
the central retail markets. In London the retailing
function of the major horticultural markets was
negligible by 1850. Several attempts were made
to establish non-specialist retail markets in various parts of London, the most notable of which
was the Baroness Burdett Coutts' Columbia Market
in the East End, but none were particularly successful.
Table 6.2 shows the proportion of produce
sold by street traders in 1851. Overall, this
amounted to approximately half of the city's fruit
requirements and a fifth of its vegetables. Costermongers seem to have concentrated their efforts
at the cheap and bulky end of the market, selling
chiefly potatoes, cabbages, onions, apples, pears
and turnips, although they were willing to buy
anything in the wholesale markets that was in season

Table 6.2: <u>The Percentage of London's Fruit and</u>
<u>Vegetables sold by Costermongers, 1851</u>

Home-grown potatoes	6.7	Home-grown apples	50.0
Imported potatoes	50.0	Imported apples	87.5
Cabbages	33.3	Home-grown pears	50.0
Broccoli and cauli-		Plums	6.7
flowers	5.0	Damsons	3.3
Turnips	10.0	Gooseberries	75.0
Carrots	3.3	Strawberries	50.0
Pears	50.0	Raspberries	5.0
Asparagus	2.5	Pineapples	10.0
Celery	12.5	Oranges	25.0
Rhubarb	10.0	Lemons	1.0
Cucumbers	12.5	Coconuts	33.3
Onions	33.3	Grapes	6.7
Watercress	46.0		

Source: H. Mayhew (1851) op. cit., 80-1.

and inexpensive. Some street traders, especially women and girls, specialized in selling one line, such as oranges or watercress. It is impossible to be certain how many street traders were involved in this trade, because the job was typically a casual form of employment. Numbers fluctuated from year to year with the vagaries of unemployment during the trade cycle, seasonally with the availability of cheap supplies of fruit and vegetables, and daily. Mayhew reported that Saturday was the costermonger's busiest day, when as many as 2,000 donkey-barrows, and over 3,000 women with shallows and head baskets visited Covent Garden alone(48).

In 1850 Spitalfields was the main market used by costermongers for purchasing their supplies, suggesting that their retail trade was largely concentrated in London's East End, where the demand for cheap vegetables was to be found, and where the development of fixed shops was retarded in the mid-nineteenth century. Evidence from later periods, however, indicates that street sales of fruit and vegetables were widespread throughout the city, both from stalls in street markets and from itinerant barrows. The relatively high proportion of fruit and vegetables sold in London's streets in 1850 dropped gradually in the late nineteenth and early twentieth centuries due to vigorous competition from the fixed shops of greengrocers and fruiterers. The numbers of these shops through time is shown in Table 6.3, where it can be seen that there were fluctuations in the shop/population

Table 6.3: London's Fruit and Vegetable Salesmen, 1817-1950

	Wholesalers (Enterprises only)	Greengrocers Central London	
		Enterprises	Branches
1817 (1)	62	-	-
1829 (2)	42	-	-
1832 (3)	131	1,147	3
1840	134	-	-
1840 (4)	79	-	-
1840 (5)	146	-	-
1845	172	-	-
1850	179	-	-
1855	214	1,116	8
1860	194	1,134	4
1865	183	1,374	18
1870	180	1,694	21
1875	204	1,723	31
1880	247	1,770	23
1885	281	1,569	21
1890	340	1,559	24
1895	400	1,477	29
1900	438	1,425	22
1905	436	1,265	21
1910	435	1,229	20
1915	444	1,112	10
1920	445	1,057	13
1925	612	1,305	20
1930	567	1,291	19
1935	554	2,227	23
1940	538	1,983	27
1945	448	1,382	27
1950	523	2,131	41

Notes:
1. Johnstone's London Commercial Guide & Street Director (1817);
2. Robson's Classification of Trades and Street Guide for London 4th ed. (1929);
3. Pigot & Co.'s National, London, & Provincial Commercial Directory for 1832-3-4 5th ed. (1832);
4. Robson's London Directory... 20th ed. (1840);
5. Pigot and Co.'s Royal National, Commercial, and Street Directory of London, for 1840 (1839);
6. 1872 data;
7. 1876 data;

120

Table 6.3: (Contd.)

Retailers

Greengrocers Suburbs		Fruiterers & Greengrocers Central London		Suburbs	
Enterprises	Branches	Enterprises	Branches	Enterprises	Branches
–	–	22	0	–	–
–	–	330	1	–	–
–	–	259	1	–	–
–	–	343	1	–	–
–	–	868	0	–	–
–	–	181	0	–	–
–	–	1,121	4	–	–
–	–	1,131	9	–	–
–	–	847	10	–	–
–	–	675	9	640	0
–	–	620	11	862	1
–	–	656	21	1,389 (6)	1
–	–	612	20	1,569 (7)	5
–	–	584	33	2,097	16
–	–	581	32	2,278 (8)	17
–	–	544	35	2,728 (9)	24
–	–	563	32	3,041 (10)	32
–	–	586	40	2,957	27
–	–	605	53	1,274	24
–	–	622	49	1,309	40
870	15	627	49	391	14
817	14	685	38	336	8
841	11	796	51	423	17
860	7	744	76	452	43
–	–	1,312	118	–	–
–	–	1,163	139	–	–
–	–	684	66	–	–
–	–	841	92	–	–

8. 1884 data;
9. 1888 data;
10. 1894 data.

Source: Post Office London and Suburban Directories,
            except where otherwise stated.

ratio. Further work is required to explain these temporal fluctuations, the evolution of the spatial pattern of outlets, and their organizational structure.

Pattern of consumption

It would be an exceptionally difficult task to estimate the demand for fruit and vegetables in the period before the First World War, requiring a full essay in its own right. The space available in this paper will be devoted to a few issues.

Supply estimates of demand are made hazardous by the intractability of the agricultural statistics. A select list of problems encountered in using this source will illustrate the point:

1. One cannot be sure before the 1920s what proportion of the vegetable crops recorded were sold for human consumption.
2. Market garden produce was recorded as a group between 1872 and 1896, but thereafter the individual crops were not listed in some cases until 1935(49).
3. Orchards were first returned in 1871, but as a double entry under both the tree crop and the under-crop. No distinction was made between dessert, culinary and vintage fruit.
4. Small-fruit statistics were collected from 1888, but were not reliable before 1897(50).
5. No record was made of the many commercial small-holdings less than one quarter of an acre in size 1869-1891, and less than one acre from 1892(51). The produce grown on allotments and in private gardens was ignored.
6. It was not until the first Census of Production in 1908 that any attempt was made to assess yields per acre. It is unsatisfactory therefore to base any discussion of fluctuations in productive capacity through time and space upon acreage statistics alone.

Demand estimates, based upon family budget information or other contemporary literary sources are similarly beset with difficulties. Fruit and vegetables are simply not mentioned in many of the budgets collected in the nineteenth century, and one cannot be sure whether this is a true indication of an absence of consumption. Allotment produce and perquisites seem to have been excluded in some cases as too infrequently available to be worth recording in the 'average' annual diet. Indeed the consumption of fruit and vegetables, at least in the period before 1914, was subject to a number of variabilities which make it difficult to quantify.

Seasonal variations in demand are well-known. They were of course especially noticeable before the era of canning and freezing dawned in the twentieth century when relatively cheap supplies of preserved fruit and vegetables became available throughout the year. The degree of seasonality can be inferred somewhat indirectly from Table 6.4 which shows the variation in monthly revenues produced by Covent Garden market.

Daily variations in the demand for food have received little attention from historians of diet. In the case of fruit and vegetables a large proportion, perhaps even the majority, of consumption was concentrated into a few meals at the weekend, well into the twentieth century. This was especially the case with fruit used in puddings and the fancier vegetables served with cooked meals.

Table 6.4: The Monthly Revenue from Covent Garden, 1870

	Rents (£)	Tolls (£)
January	629.45	308.14
February	520.50	277.82
March	548.08	362.55
April	643.80	408.77
May	560.10	402.89
June	564.55	777.30
July	669.40	1,086.71
August	555.60	803.34
September	541.55	638.49
October	629.40	505.71
November	528.88	396.83
December	637.38	369.75

Source: Greater London Record Office (London Records): E/BER/CG/E/10/52.

Most fruits and many of the choicer vegetables were considered luxury items by consumers throughout the period 1850-1950. This helps to explain the upsurge of demand in the late nineteenth century as the standard of living of the mass of the people improved with increased real wages. It also suggests that there is likely to have been a high income-elasticity of demand on the more expensive produce. We have very little evidence before the First World War to confirm this, however, beyond the sort of crude aggregate data portrayed in Table 6.5, and this means that any estimates of 'average' demand cannot adequately take account of the wide range of demand among different socio-economic groups. Another area of neglect in British dietary history has been the regional variability of food intake. It is true that data are scanty and unreliable, but we should at least ask some pertinent questions of the information that is available. Table 6.6 is a compilation of the sort of data that must be pressed into service if regional variations in preferences for individual items within the broad category of fruit and vegetables are to be described.

A final variability that demands attention is secular change through time in the population's dietary habits. Mayhew's London data show a fruit and vegetable diet biased towards the less perishable bulky commodities, but we know that tastes changed in the period 1850-1950 because we can make a comparison with the results of the National Food Survey. Table 6.7 indicates that by the late-twentieth century there had been a dramatic reduction in the quantity consumed of heavy vegetables such as cabbage, turnips, cauliflowers and onions, and a correspondingly sharp increase in purchases of peas, beans, cucumbers, lettuce, apples and grapes. Some items were new to the list, including pineapples, tomatoes, bananas and brussels sprouts.

Conclusion

This paper has sketched the outline of the production and supply system of the horticultural trade from 1850 to 1950. No attempt has been made to estimate the supplies of fruit and vegetables available for consumption in this period for a number of reasons. First, several estimates have been published at the aggregate level of the nation which do not require repetition here(52). Second, a great deal more detailed research into the agricultural statistics, changing yield patterns, and import/export data is necessary before refinements are possible at this national scale. Thirdly, the present author is sceptical anyway of the utility of estimates of this sort because of the variabilities in consumption patterns with social

Table 6.5: The Variability of Demand for Fruit and Vegetables with income

(a) Board of Trade Survey of 1944 urban working-men's families in Britain (1904):

Average weekly income (shillings per family)

Weekly expenditure per family (d)	0-25 (d)	25-30 (d)	30-35 (d)	35-40 (d)	40< (d)
Fruit and vegetables	4.69	6.85	10.09	11.76	15.53
Potatoes	8.64	9.62	10.30	10.15	9.98

(b) 1152 family budgets (1932-5):

Average weekly income (shillings per head)

Weekly expenditure per head (d)	0.10 (d)	10-15 (d)	15-20 (d)	20-30 (d)	30-45 (d)	45-< (d)
Fruit	2.4	4.6	6.6	9.5	13.0	20.0
Potatoes	2.5	2.9	3.0	3.0	3.1	3.0
Other vegetables	1.5	2.6	3.9	5.2	6.5	8.5

Source: (a) Board of Trade, Second Series of Memoranda, Statistical Tables and Charts ..., Parliamentary Papers 1905 (Cd.2337) LXXXIV, pp. 15-44;

(b) J.B. Orr, Food, Health and Income (2nd ed, London, 1937), p. 74.

Table 6.6: Regional Demand for Various Canned Fruits
and Vegetables as Demonstrated by the
Percentage of Shops in Each Area Carrying
Stocks (1931-2)

(a) Fruit (Survey of 1343 retail grocers)

	London and South (%)	Mid- lands (%)	Lanca- shire (%)	York- shire (%)	Glasgow (%)
Peaches	100	100	100	100	100
Pears	99	100	100	100	100
Apricots	97	98	94	98	75
Fruit Salad	83	87	68	89	81
Loganberries	44	55	18	30	8
Strawberries	21	52	25	56	18
Plums	28	48	23	25	11
Damsons	4	17	21	8	-

(b) Vegetables (Survey of 583 retail grocers)

	London (%)	Birming- ham (%)	Liver- pool (%)	N.E. Coast (%)
Baked Beans	99	99	100	100
Peas	97	100	94	96
Tomatoes	92	99	97	98
Asparagus	46	23	19	24
Sweet Corn	17	2	8	8
Spinach	10	2	6	11
Carrots	3	-	3	4

Source: (a) Empire Marketing Board, The Demand
for Canned Fruit (London, 1931),
p. 12;

(b) Empire Marketing Board, The Demand
for Canned Vegetables (London, 1932),
p. 10.

Table 6.7: A Comparison of the Demand for Selected Fruits and Vegetables in London in 1851 and 1978

(Quantities in lbs per head per annum)

Fruit	1851* (lb)	1978+ (lb)
Apples	15.48	26.78
Pears	7.96	3.12
Oranges	7.34	12.97
Bananas	-	12.55
Stone Fruit	5.68	3.64
Grapes	0.50	1.66
Soft fruit, other than grapes	8.22	2.37
Rhubarb	1.74	1.76
Nuts	4.22	1.76
Dried fruit	17.99	3.51

Vegetables		
Potatoes	148.64	130.39
Cabbages	68.33	21.03
Broccoli and Cauliflowers	27.29	8.71
Turnips and Swedes	40.84	2.31
Carrots	6.87	11.28
Peas	3.34	15.67
Beans	2.28	18.56
Lettuce	1.71	5.53
Onions	31.82	13.20
Cucumbers	0.04	4.32
Tomatoes	-	18.82
Brussels Sprouts	-	8.52

Notes: * Allowing 10 per cent for wastage in wholesale markets and in retailing, and assuming that no fruit and vegetables were exported from London at this date.

+ Fresh produce only, except for preserved and processed potatoes, nuts, dried fruit, peas, beans and tomatoes, all of which are included.

Source: H. Mayhew (1851), op.cit.; Ministry of Agriculture, Household Food Consumption and Expenditure: 1978. Annual Report of the National Food Survey Committee (1980), pp. 45-7.

class and region discussed above. Emphasis was put rather upon geographical and structural evolution of the trade, in the hope that future work may build upon this foundation and elucidate the link between the availability of supplies and changing patterns of demand. London had the country's most sophisticated supply system in 1850, and benefited most rapidly from the technical and organizational improvements of the late Victorian period. The result, one suspects, although no reliable confirmatory evidence is to hand, was a very different dietary pattern in terms of fruit and vegetables, and possibly also other foodstuffs, from the other cities and rural areas of Britain(53). The question arises, therefore, whether the regional variations in consumption observable in the past, and in many cases surviving to the present day, were mainly a result of the differing pace at which local areas were able to develop the production of their own fruit and vegetables, or the creation of the structures necessary to import the produce of other regions. An answer must await the results of the regional studies of relationships between local conditions of production, supply and consumption which are urgently needed.

NOTES

1. For a modern interpretation of von Thünen's model see W.C. Found, A Theoretical Approach to Land-Use Patterns (1971).
2. P. Hall (ed.), Von Thünen's Isolated State (Oxford, 1966), p. 9.
3. G.B.G. Bull, 'The Changing Landscape of Rural Middlesex', unpublished Ph.D. thesis, University of London (1957); D.W. Harvey, 'Aspects of Agriculture and Rural Change in Kent, 1800-1900', unpublished Ph.D. thesis, University of Cambridge (1971); A.G. Parton, 'Town and Country in Surrey, c. 1800-1870: a Study in Historical Geography',unpublished Ph.D. thesis, University of Hull (1973).
4. G.B.G. Bull, 'Thomas Milne's Land Utilisation Map of the London Area in 1800', Geographical Journal, 122 (1957), pp. 25-30; E.C. Willatts, 'Land Utilisation in Middlesex in the past', in L.D. Stamp (ed.), The Land of Britain, Part 79 (1937), pp. 294-5; G.B.G. Bull, 'Thomas Milne's Land Use Map of London and Environs in 1800', London Topographical Society

publications, nos. 118 and 119 (1975-6); R.J.P. Kain, 'The London Topographical Society's Edition of Thomas Milne's Map of London', Bulletin of the Society of University Cartographers, 13 (1979), pp. 16-22.

5. J. Cuthill, Market Gardening, or the Various Methods Adopted by Gardeners in Growing for the London Markets (1851).

6. C. Whitehead, 'The Cultivation of Hops, Fruit and Vegetables', Journal of the Royal Agricultural Society of England, series 2, 14 (1878), p. 750.

7. H. Evershed, 'Market-gardening', J.R. Ag.S.E. series 2, 7 (1871), p. 423.

8. L.G. Bennett, 'The Development and Present Structure of the Horticultural Industry in Middlesex and the London Region', unpublished Ph.D. thesis, University of Reading (1950).

9. P.G. Atherall, 'The Displacement of Market Gardening around London by Urban Growth from 1745-1939', unpublished M. Litt. thesis, University of Cambridge (1975).

10. C. Whitehead, op.cit. pp. 749-52.

11. C.W. Shaw, The London Market Gardens (1979).

12. This pattern does not seem to have developed to the same extent around other British cities where consumption was on an altogether different scale.

13. C. Whitehead, 'Hints on Vegetable and Fruit Farming', J.R.Ag.S.E., series 2, 18 (1882), p. 74.

14. C. Whitehead, 'Fruit-Farming in Kent', Journal of the Bath and West of England Society, series 3, 15 (1883-4), pp. 150-77; W.E. Bear, 'Flower and Fruit Farming in England, III; Fruit Growing in the Open', J.R.Ag.S.E., series 3, 10 (1899), pp. 30-86; D.W. Harvey, 'Fruit Growing in Kent in the Nineteenth Century', Archaeologia Cantiana, 79 (1964), pp. 95-108.

15. Fruit and vegetable production in Wales and Scotland never reached a level of national significance except, perhaps, for soft fruit at Blairgowrie.

16. R.R.W. Folley, Intensive Crop Economics: an Outline of the Principles of Resource Use, Management and Marketing as Adapted for Horticultural Crops (1973), p. 78.

17. Ministry of Agriculture and Fisheries, Horticulture in Britain, Part 1: Vegetables (1967), p. 13.

18. R.R.W. Folley (1973), op.cit. p. 78.

19. K.M. Round, 'Celery Growing in the Fens', Agriculture, 67 (1960), pp. 189-91.
20. J. Tasker, 'The West Riding Rhubarb Industry', Agriculture, 59 (1953), pp. 386-91.
21. J.T. Coppock, An Agricultural Geography of Great Britain (1971), pp. 279-80.
22. J. Udale, 'Market Gardening and Fruit Growing in the Vale of Evesham', J.R.Ag.S.E., 69 (1908), pp. 95-104; R.S. Lodge, 'The Horticulture of the Vale of Evesham', unpublished Ph.D. thesis, University of Birmingham (1972); G.M. Robinson, 'Late Victorian Agriculture in the Vale of Evesham', School of Geography University of Oxford, Research Paper 16 (1976).
23. F. Beavington, 'The Change to more Extensive Methods of Market Gardening in Bedfordshire', Transactions of the Institute of British Geographers, 33 (1963), pp. 89-100; idem, 'Early Market Gardening in Bedfordshire', Trans. I.B.G. 37 (1965), pp. 91-100; idem, 'The Development of Market Gardening in Bedfordshire, 1799-1939', Agricultural History Review, 23 (1975), pp. 23-47; R. Webber, 'Early Market Gardening at Sandy', Bedfordshire Magazine, 14 (1974), pp. 146-9.
24. E.A. Pratt, The Transition in Agriculture, (1906), p. 116; A.D. Hall, A Pilgrimage of British Farming (1913), p. 341; H.M. Cole, 'An Economic Study of the Broccoli Crop in West Cornwall', University of Bristol, Department of Economics (Agricultural Economics), Report no. 89 (1958).
25. C.A. Wheadon, 'The History and Cultivation of the Tomato in Guernsey', La Société Guernesiaise, Reports and Transactions, 12 (1935), pp. 337-50; M.G. Harwood, 'Tomato Growing Prior to 1940', Review of the Guernsey Society, 33 (1977), pp. 9-13.
26. G.J. Gleed, 'The Strawberry Industry of South Hampshire', J.R.Ag.S.E., 92 (1931), pp. 201-13; E. Thomas and G. Bissett, 'The Strawberry Industry of South Hampshire', University of Reading Agricultural Economics Department, Bulletin, 45 (1933).
27. W.S. Mansfield, 'Notable Farming Enterprises II: the Farms of Messrs Chivers & Sons, Ltd., Histon, Cambridgeshire', J.R.Ag.S.E. 92 (1931) pp. 142-51; E.A. Pratt, op.cit. pp. 43-7.
28. W.L. Hinton, 'Distribution of Horticultural Output in England and Wales', Agriculture, 67 (1960), pp. 184-8; J.T. Coppock, An Agri-

cultural Atlas of England and Wales (1964), pp. 118-54; R. Webber, Market Gardening: the History of Commercial Flowers, Fruit and Vegetable Growing (Newton Abbot, 1975), pp. 151-85.

29. W.E. Bear, 'Flower and Fruit Farming in England, IV: Fruit Growing under Glass', J.R.Ag.S.E. series 3, 10 (1899), pp. 267-313.

30. P.E. Cross, 'The Extension of Market Gardening into Agriculture', Journal of the Royal Society of Arts, 91 (1943), pp. 310-18; R.H. Best and R.M. Gasson, 'The Changing Location of Intensive Crops', Wye College, University of London, Studies in Rural Land Use, 6 (1966), p. 71.

31. Ministry of Agriculture (1967), op.cit. pp. 42-5.

32. (A. Wynter), 'The London Commissariat', Quarterly Review, 190 (1854), p. 302.

33. In 1888 32 local growers paid for annual wagon stands and an average of 166 wagons used the casual stands per day: First Report of the Royal Commission on Market Rights and Tolls, vol. II Parliamentary Papers 1888 (c. 5550-1) LIII, p. 433, QQ. 4258-60.

34. P.P. 1839 VIII, Q. 156.

35. The most comprehensive and detailed account of vegetable marketing during this period is given in Ministry of Agriculture and Fisheries, Vegetable Marketing in England and Wales, Economic Series, 25 (1935).

36. L.G. Bennett, 'The Marketing of Horticultural Produce Grown in Bedfordshire, West Cornwall, Wisbech and the Lea Valley', University of Reading, Department of Agricultural Economics, Miscellaneous Studies, 12 (1957), pp. 27-8.

37. R.J. Battersby, 'The Development of Market Gardening in England, 1850-1914', unpublished Ph.D. thesis, University of London (1960), p. 135.

38. Ibid. p. 156.

39. Report of the Committee on Horticultural Marketing P.P. 1956-7 (Cmnd. 61) IX, p. 258.

40. Showcase Publicity Co. Ltd., Fruit, Vegetable and Flower Markets of England: Borough Market (1954), p. 83.

41. L.G. Bennett (1957), op.cit.

42. Departmental Committee on Distribution and Prices of Agricultural Produce: Interim Report

on Fruit and Vegetables P.P. 1923 (Cmd. 1892) IX, p. 19.

43. Report of the Imperial Economic Committee on Marketing and Preparing for Market of Foodstuffs Produced in the Overseas Ports of the Empire. Third Report: Fruit P.P. 1926 (Cmd. 2658) XII, p. 25.

44. G. Dodd, The Food of London, (1856), ch. 10; Royal Commission on Market Rights and Tolls, Vol. II, P.P. 1888 (c.5550-1) LIII, pp. 116-172; London County Council, Public Control Department, London Markets: Special Report ... (1893); W.W. Glenny, 'The Fruit and Vegetable Markets of the Metropolis', J.R.Ag.S.E. series 3, 7 (1896), pp. 53-67; Fourth Report of the Departmental Committee on the Wholesale Markets of London: London Wholesale Fruit and Vegetable Markets. P.P. 1921 (Cmd. 1341) XII: C. Maughan, Markets of London (1931) pp. 157-75; W.J. Passingham, London's Markets: their Origin and History (1935) pp. 56-127; Ministry of Agriculture, Markets and Fairs in England and Wales Part VI: London Markets, Economic Series, 26 (1930).

45. J. Hunt, Covent Garden Market (1926); Fantus Co., Study for the Relocation of Covent Garden Market (1963); R. Webber, Covent Garden: Mud Salad Market (1969); London County Council, Survey of London, vol. XXXVI: The Parish of St. Paul Covent Garden (1970), R. Thorne, Covent Garden Market (London, 1980); P.J. Atkins, 'Covent Garden and the Food of London', unpublished paper read at the Museum of London (June, 1980).

46. J. Page, 'The Sources of Supply of the Manchester Fruit and Vegetable Market',J.R.Ag.S.E. series 2, 16 (1880), pp. 475-85.

47. W.E. Bear, 'The Food Supply of Manchester, I: Vegetable Produce', J.R.Ag.S.E. series 3, 8(1897), pp. 205-28.

48. H. Mayhew (1851), op.cit. p. 81.

49. W.F. Darke, 'A Short Guide to Pre-War English Outdoor Vegetable Statistics', Journal of the Royal Statistical Society, 105 (1942), pp. 328-35.

50. R.H. Rew, Head of the Statistical Branch of the Board of Agriculture, in evidence before the Departmental Committee ... on the Fruit Industry..., P.P. 1905 (Cd 2589) XX p.8,Q30.

51. Ministry of Agriculture, A Century of Agricultural Statistics, Great Britain 1866-1966

(London, 1968), p. 7.

52. Notably J.P. Greaves and D.F. Hollingsworth, 'Trends in Food Consumption in the United Kingdom', World Review of Nutrition and Dietetics, 6 (1966), pp. 38-9; D.J. Oddy, 'The Working Class Diet, 1886-1914', unpublished Ph.D. thesis, University of London (1971), Ch. 7.

53. The diet of 'the average Londoner', however, probably masks as great a variation of consumption due to socio-economic and ethnic differences as does that of 'the average Briton'.

7. THE NUTRITIONAL IMPORTANCE OF FRUIT AND VEGETABLES

A.E. BENDER

Fruit and vegetables play an important but very variable role in the diet. They are the major, and in many instances the only sources of vitamin C. They supply a large part of the vitamin A as carotene: some supply thiamin. Others are good sources of iron and calcium. However, they differ so much from one another in their nutrients that it is not really possible to group them together as is usually done in textbooks of nutrition. Such groupings as are used appear to be culinary rather than botanical or nutritional. For example tomatoes and cucumbers which botanically are fruits are classed as vegetables; celery (a petiole) as a vegetable while rhubarb, also a petiole, is classed as a fruit. Olives, and avocado pears are rarely mentioned. It would seem that sweet foods, such as the melon, or foods usually eaten after sweetening, such as rhubarb, are classed as fruits, otherwise as exemplified by courgettes, pumpkins and cucumbers (the same family as the melon) and tomato, as vegetables. This is all usually taken for granted under the approach 'you know what I mean' - and usually one does, but nutritionally each must be considered on its merits.

Carotene

This is the one nutrient that makes itself visible in fruits like apricots and peaches and particularly in the carrot (and, incidentally, in the yellow as distinct from white maize). This has led to grouping together yellow and orange fruits and vegetables but even this is inadequate since melons, mangoes and papaya can range from a trace of carotene (very pale colour) to as much as 1,000 micrograms per 100 g, and carrots can

134

vary from 90 to 3,600 micrograms per 100 g (the recommended daily intake for an adult is 750 micrograms). Carotene is present in all green vegetables but its colour is masked by the chlorophyll. Even there the amounts vary with the depth of green colour - the outer deep green leaves are richer in carotene, and also in vitamin K and folic acid, than the inner white leaves.

Vitamin C

A shortage of vitamin C gives rise to scurvy and the importance of fruits as a source of this vitamin came to light in the eighteenth century. Dr. J. Lind showed that scurvy could be prevented or cured with oranges and lemons; Captain Cook was able to spend 3 years away from his home base by taking fruits and vegetables on board at every port; and even before then, Cartier in 1535 learned to make an extract of spruce tips to prevent scurvy. During the fifteenth and sixteenth centuries scurvy was certainly common throughout Europe since fruits and vegetables were little cultivated and there was no method of preserving them to retain the vitamin. The poor vitamin C status of those on land is illustrated by the case in the Plymouth magistrate's court in 1878. The captain of the Chyrolite was fined 40 shillings (the minimum) for not taking on board sufficient lime juice during a trip from Cardiff to Aden - when the supplies were finished scurvy broke out. We now know that the average well-fed person can go without vitamin C for about 5 months before his reserves fail, so the sailors who got scurvy as soon as the supplies of lime juice gave out must have been in a poor state before they left land, and the lime juice, of course, must have been nearly devoid of vitamin C. We now know that the vitamin C in fruit juice is rapidly oxidised when exposed to the air.

Even today, potatoes supply on average one-quarter of the vitamin C intake, and in winter as much as one-half. The winter problem is aggravated by the loss of vitamin C from potatoes during storage - the level falls from about 30 mg per 100 g when harvested to 8-10 mg in Spring.

Although fruits and vegetables are sources of vitamin C they differ considerably from one another in the amount present; Table 7.1 shows that vegetables can vary from as little as 6 mg to 100 mg and fruits can cover an even wider range,

Table 7.1: <u>The composition of Vegetables</u>

Composition - per 100 g food (raw unless otherwise stated)

	Calcium (mg)	Iron (mg)
Leafy Vegetables		
cabbage savoy	75	0.9
winter	57	0.6
sprouts	32	0.7
broccoli tops	100	1.5
endive	44	2.8
lettuce	23	0.9
spinach (boiled)	600	4.0
watercress	220	1.6
Flowers		
cauliflower	21	0.5
globe artichoke (boiled)	44	0.5
Roots		
onions	31	0.3
turnips	59	0.1
radishes	44	1.9
carrots	48	0.6
beet	25	0.4
Parsnips	55	0.6
potatoes	8	0.5
Stems		
asparagus (boiled)	26	0.9
celery	52	0.6
rhubarb	100	0.4
Recommended Daily Intakes (Adult Male)		
10% RDI	50	1
20% RDI	100	2

Table 7.1: (Contd.)

Riboflavin (mg)	Thiamin (mg)	Vitamin C (mg)	Vitamin A (ug)
0.05	0.06	60	50
0.05	0.06	55	50
(0.15)	0.10	90	70
0.15	0.10	110	400
0.10	0.06	12	330
0.08	0.07	15	160
0.15	0.07	25	1,000
0.10	0.10	60	500
0.10	0.10	60	5
0.03	0.07	8	15
0.05	0.03	10	0
0.05	0.04	25	0
0.02	0.04	25	0
0.05	0.06	6	2,000
0.05	0.03	6	0
0.08	0.10	15	0
0.04	0.1	8-20	0
0.08	0.10	20	80
0.03	0.03	7	0
0.03	0.01	10	10
0.18	0.13	3	75
0.36	0.26	6	150

3 - 200 mg, and in the case of the West Indian cherry to as much as 3,000 mg per 100 g. This is in the raw state and a great deal is lost in cooking. The danger of generalizing about these foods is illustrated by the statement in the text-book by Davidson, Passmore, Truswell and Brock that 'a single helping of vegetables - 90 g - even if it has been badly treated by the cook, will usually provide at least 10 mg of ascorbic acid, an amount known to prevent scurvy'(1). This is far from true. Chick and Dalyell(2) reported that despite a good supply of vegetables 40 out of 64 children in a hospital in Vienna developed scurvy. They showed that 70 per cent was lost after cooking for 20 minutes at 100° C (not an inordinate length of time according to current institutional methods) and 90 per cent was lost after 60 minutes at 60-70° C. Fifty years later we found that some potatoes served in school meals were completely devoid of vitamin C, with the average content of 1.6 mg per 100 g, and cabbage could be as low as 1.3 mg (average 10.1 mg/100g)(3).

Vegetables

Three major textbooks, two American and one British, were consulted for classifying of vegetables; all three grouped them into leafy, flowering and root vegetables. Table 7.1 shows the nutrient content of a number of these taken from the standard Food Composition Tables(4). Three caveats must be entered. First, the iron and calcium are poorly absorbed from most foods and to a very variable extent, to the present discussion is restricted to the total amount present in the food. Secondly, since vitamin C can be destroyed by cooking only values for raw foods, i.e. the maximum possible, are given, except for three foods where the raw food is not included in the tables. Thirdly, there is a great variation in the nutrient content of plants depending on variety, soil, climate and growing conditions, so the values quoted are averages of a wide range.

There is no accepted method of classing foods into 'rich', 'good' and 'fair' sources of nutrients. One method is to relate the nutrient concentration to the energy supplied, so that a food or dish supplying 10 per cent of the energy might be des-cribed as a good source of a nutrient if it supplied 10 per cent of that nutrient. More than 10 per cent could be considered a 'rich source' and less correspondingly 'poor'.

Since most, but by no means all, fruits and vegetables make an insignificant contribution to the energy intake this method is not applicable. Instead, as an arbitrary distinction, a food may be considered to be a reasonable source of the nutrient if 100 g, an average portion, supplies 10 per cent of the recommended daily intake and a good source if the same amount supplies 20 per cent of the Recommended Daily Intake(RDI).

Among the three textbooks consulted that of Krause and Mahan(5) describes green, leafy vegetables as being 'important' sources of calcium, iron and riboflavin. Briggs and Calloway(6) describe them as being 'especially rich' in calcium and iron. Davidson et al(7) state less specifically that most vegetables contain amounts of calcium and iron 'that are probably physiologically signifi- cant' and more specifically 'that many leafy vegetables are "rich" in calcium and that their iron is well absorbed because of the presence of vitamin C, and that most leafy vegetables are "fair" sources of riboflavin.' Table 7.1 shows that on the basis outlined above five of the eight leafy vegetables are reasonable sources of calcium and three are rich sources. Four are sources of iron but only two are rich sources. The statements that they are good or even fair sources of ribo- flavin are completely incorrect - not one of the leafy vegetables supplies even 10 per cent of the RDI. Krause and Mahan(8) describe flowering vegetables as good sources of iron and riboflavin and root vegetables, in general, as good sources of thiamin, but these statements are incorrect.

Contribution to the diet

The contribution made by a food towards the total diet obviously depends on the amount eaten as well as the nutrient concentration. It is well known, for example, that although potatoes are not rich sources of vitamin C and thiamin they make an important contribution since they are eaten in relatively large amounts - and, indeed, make an appreciable contribution to the energy and protein intakes as well, even in the mixed diets commonly eaten in Great Britain and the United States. As distinct from the concentrations given in Table 7.1, Table 7.2 shows the contributions made to the diet by fruits and vegetables. In the U.K. they supply 10 per cent of the energy

Table 7.2: Contribution to the average intake of nutrients from fruit and vegetables (per cent total)

United Kingdom

	Energy (%)	Protein (%)	Iron (%)	Vit.C (%)	B1 (%)	B2 (%)	A (%)
Potatoes	4.7	3.4	6.2	26	9	2.7	
Leafy & salad vegetables			1.8	10	1	1.5	1
Tomatoes				6			1
Carrots							14
All vegetables	7.5	8.6	17.2	55	16	8	20
All fruits	2.4	1.0	3.6	33	3	2	1
Total	10	10	21	88	19	10	20

United States

	Energy (%)	Protein (%)	Iron (%)	Vit.C (%)	B1 (%)	B2 (%)	A (%)
All vegetables	5.6	6	15	40	12	7	43
All fruits	3	1.1	4.1	40	4.5	2	7
Total	9	7	20	80	17	9	50

Note: Contributions <10 omitted.
Source: U.K.: National Food Survey (1977); U.S.A.: U.S. Department of Agriculture, National Food Review (1978).

and of the protein; largely due to potatoes. As might be expected fruits and vegetables provide nearly all the vitamin C of both the American and British diets; together with 20 per cent of the thiamin, (half coming from potato) and 10 per cent of the riboflavin.

The difference between the individual foods is further illustrated by the enormous contribution made by one food, the carrot, to the total vitamin A intake in the U.K. - 14 per cent.

Since British people are among the lowest consumers of fruits and vegetables in Europe it is surprising to find that these foods make similar contributions to the American diet. The one major difference is that they provide 20 per cent of the vitamin A in the U.K. diet and 50 per cent in the U.S. diet. This may partly be due to methods of calculation and partly to the contribution, 5 per cent, made by the sweet potato in the U.S. whereas it is not included in the British diet. Briggs and Calloway state that the calcium is unavailable (to what extent is not stated) in spinach, chard, sorrel, parsley and beet greens but that the others 'rank next to milk in sources of calcium'. In the same publication it is shown that dairy products provide 74.6 per cent of the average U.S. intake of calcium while fruits and vegetables combined provide only 9.6 per cent(9).

Energy and protein

Fruits and vegetables are regarded as being very low in energy content and for some of them, particularly the leafy vegetables and the stems; this is true since they are largely water and cellulose. Indeed their bulky nature and low energy density allows them to be eaten relatively freely by those on weight-reducing diets. However, the root crops and underground storage organs (tubers and rhizomes) are a more concentrated source of energy and, indeed, potatoes and yams which are the staple food in some communities, provide respectively 80 and 120 kcal per 100 g when cooked. Some of the fruits, as mentioned later, are con- centrated sources of energy.

Protein content can be calculated either per 100 g of food or as a proportion of the total energy content of the food. The latter is the more informa- tive since the former method can give rise to apparent changes in composition on cooking. An extreme example is rice; this gains two volumes of water when cooked so apparently falls in protein calculated per 100 g weight of the food, but there is no change when calculated as protein energy per 100 kcal of total energy.

Table 7.3 shows that some vegetables gain water on cooking and so provide less energy per 100 g - the energy content of marrow falls to half, that of potatoes, sweet potatoes, onions and turnips falls a little. Other vegetables lose water and so have increased energy per 100 g, such as plantain and parsnip. Table 7.3 also illustrates that these foods cannot be grouped together nutritionally. Leafy vegetables are described as poor sources of energy but range from 8 kcal per 100 g for sea-kale to 30 kcal for spinach (boiled). However, the protein content of spinach is exceptionally high. At 5.1 per cent of the wet weight of cooked spinach it is about half that of cereals, and about three times as great as most of the other leafy vegetables. On an energy basis all the leafy vegetables provide exceptionally large proportions of proteins - ranging from 35 per cent for lettuce to 86 per cent for watercress: marrow, cucumber and green peppers are similar. However, the realistic measure here is the amount eaten and 100 g may be considered a reasonable portion - so supplying only 2-5 grams of protein. So far as the root crops are concerned portions may be larger than this, possibly 100-200 g for the side dish in western diets for foods such as parsnips, swedes and carrots, up to 300-500 grams for potatoes so supplying up to 400 kcal (1700 kJ) - but still only 7 g of protein. Only when foods such as potatoes and yams become the staple food are they eaten in sufficient amounts to supply reasonable amounts of protein. Plantains are exceptional in being so low in protein, 1 per cent on a weight basis and only 3.4 per cent of the energy. So even if they are eaten in amounts sufficient to satisfy energy requirements they do not supply enough protein.

Several points of interest arise among the fruits. When dried they are, of course, much more concentrated but when they are rehydrated by the usual soaking and boiling they do not regain all the water lost from the fresh fruit, and so stewed figs and apricots, for example, are about three times as concentrated as the fresh, wet, version. Dried dates are another staple. They are sufficiently concentrated in energy to provide a large part of the diet without having to be consumed in unacceptable bulk - 500 g provides 1250 kcal (5.3 MJ), about half the daily needs but they are poor sources of protein at 3.4 per cent. So an intake sufficient to provide half the day's energy would provide less than one third of the protein. On this basis figs are superior; they are slightly lower in energy and are twice as rich as dates in protein.

Olives and avocado pears, are two fruits so high in their fat content, and so are unusual among these foods, that they are highly concentrated sources of energy. Legumes are omitted from this discussion since they lie outside the topic of this chapter. They differ from the fruits and vegetables under discussion since they are major sources of protein, energy and other nutrients in many diets.

Other factors

Dietary fibre is the name given to the indigestible parts of plant foods and includes cellulose and hemicellulose found in vegetables and cereals, and pectin found in fruits. It has been shown in recent years to have beneficial effects on bowel disorders but again, it is not possible to generalize about the different foods. Apart from the finding that cereal bran fibre is the most useful form of dietary fibre physiologically, the materials present in fruits and vegetables differ in type and amount. Cummings et al(10) showed that carrot had no effect on intestinal transit time (a measure of the physiological effect) while the same amount of dietary fibre from cabbage and apple did have an effect, although very much less than that of cereal bran. Furthermore, the amounts of fibre differ in the different foods.

Sodium and potassium are concerned with water balance in the body; potassium is present mainly inside the cells and sodium, together with chloride, is outside i.e. in the extracellular water. Too high an intake of sodium is regarded as being one of the factors involved in high blood pressure, which in turn, is associated with many of the diseases of western society. Fruits and vegetables are low in their content of sodium and so are recommended for people on low-sodium diets. Moreover, they are richer in potassium than sodium and this is considered to be of benefit. This appears to be the basis of the popular belief in

Table 7.3: Energy and protein content of fruit and vegetables

Food	Energy (per 100g)		Protein	
	kcal	kJ	(g/100g)	(% energy)
Leafy vegetables				
cabbage, winter, raw	22	92	2.8	53
boiled	15	66	1.7	47
lettuce	12	51	1.0	35
spinach, boiled	30	128	5.1	71
spring greens, boiled	10	43	1.7	71
seakale, boiled	8	33	1.4	74
watercress, raw	14	61	2.9	86
Root crops				
carrots, raw	23	98	0.7	12.6
boiled	19	79	0.6	13.2
onions, raw	23	99	0.9	16.5
boiled	13	53	0.6	19.2
swedes, raw	21	88	1.1	21.9
boiled	18	76	0.9	21
turnips, raw	20	86	0.8	16.5
boiled	14	60	0.7	20.8
parsnips, raw	49	210	1.7	14.5
boiled	56	238	1.3	10
potatoes, raw	87	372	2.1	10.1 x
boiled	80	343	1.4	7.4 x
(chipped, fried)	253	1065	3.8	6.3
yam, raw	131	560	2.0	6.4
	119	508	1.6	5.6
sweet potatoes, raw	91	387	1.2	5.5
boiled	85	363	1.1	5.4
Vegetable/fruits				
peppers, green	15	65	0.9	25
marrow, raw	16	69	0.6	15.6 x
boiled	7	29	0.4	24.3 x
plantain, raw	112	477	1.0	3.8
boiled	122	518	1.0	3.4

FRUIT, VEGETABLES AND NUTRITION

Table 7.3:(Contd.)

Food	Energy (per 100g)		Protein	
	kcal	kJ	(g/100g)	(% energy)
Vegetable/fruits contd.				
cucumber	10	43	0.6	25
olives (in brine)	103	422	0.9	3.7
avocado pear	223	922	4.2	7.9
Fruits				
apples	46	196	0.3	2.8
apricots, fresh	28	117	0.6	8.9
dried	182	776	4.8	11
stewed *	66	288	1.8	11.4
cherries	47	201	0.6	5.3
grapes	61	258	0.6	4.1
pears	41	175	0.3	3.2
peaches	37	156	0.6	6.8
bananas	79	337	1.1	5.8
dates (dried)	248	1056	2.0	3.4
figs, fresh	41	174	1.3	13.2
dried	213	908	3.6	7
stewed *	118	504	2.0	7

Note: x   differential loss of carbohydrate and protein in
         cooking

   *   dried fruit stewed without adding sugar

145

Switzerland and Germany in the health-giving properties of apple juice - its high ratio of potassium to sodium is believed to be of general benefit to health. Apart from their content of dietary fibre which helps to maintain bowel function, fruits contain substances that stimulate intestinal muscles. Prunes, for example, contain hydroxyphenyl isatin which stimulates the smooth muscle of the colon and has long been used together with 'syrup of figs' as a laxative.

Some of the vegetables when raw contain small amounts of toxins; the brassica family contain goitrogens but the amounts ingested in the normal diet are readily dealt with by the body. Similarly rhubarb contains oxalic acid (5 lb contains a lethal amount) but the amounts normally consumed are rapidly excreted. Fruits contain a varied range of acids, malic in apples, plums and tomatoes, benzoic in cranberries, tartaric in grapes, oxalic in strawberries, rhubarb and spinach. The small amounts eaten are, as stated, not toxic but may interfere with the absorption of iron, calcium and possibly other mineral salts by combining with them to form insoluble and so unabsorbed compounds such as calcium oxalate and iron phosphate. The problems have not been clarified but explain why the calcium in foods like spinach, rich in oxalate, are probably more poorly absorbed than the calcium from other foods. Since oxalate and phosphate can render iron salts insoluble and reduce their absorption, while vitamin C aids the absorption of iron from foods, the whole question of the availability of minerals from fruits and vegetables presents a complicated problem to the nutritionist.

NOTES

1. S. Davidson, R. Passmore, J.F. Brock and A.S. Truswell, Human Nutrition and Dietetics 7th ed. (1979).
2. H. Chick and E.J. Dalyell, British Medical Journal, 9 Oct. 1920.
3. A.E. Bender, M.C. Harris and A. Getreuer, British Medical Journal 1, pp. 757-9.
4. A.A. Paul and D.A.T. Southgate, The Composition of Foods, M.R.C., S.R. No. 297 (1978).
5. M.V. Krause and L.K. Mahan, Food, Nutrition and Diet Therapy 6th ed. (1979).
6. G.M. Briggs and D.H. Calloway, Nutrition and Physical Fitness (Philadelphia, 1979).
7. Davidson et al, op.cit.

8. Krause and Mahan, op.cit.
9. Briggs and Calloway, op.cit. p. 398.
10. J.H. Cummings, D.A.T. Southgate et al, Lancet
     1, pp. 5-9.

8. INFANT FEEDING, SANITATION AND DIARRHOEA IN COLLIERY COMMUNITIES, 1880-1911

IAN BUCHANAN

Introduction

This article concerns itself with infant mortality from the diarrhoeal group of diseases, over the turn of the century. Its objective is to achieve an understanding of the causes of this mortality, through a close consideration of local experiences. To this end infant mortality is examined in six coal mining communities. These are Aberdare and Rhondda in Glamorgan, Wigan and Hindley in Lancashire, and Hetton-le-Hole and Houghton-le-Spring in Durham(1). It is contended that the bulk of deaths from this important group formed an etiological entity. That is, that the disease involved shared common causes which contribute to an understanding of the mortality. Specifically, it is argued that they may be understood in terms of a complex interaction involving urban insanitation and the method of infant feeding adopted, and that the common house fly was an important infective agent.

By the end of the Edwardian era three main causes of death were directly associated with artificial feeding and insanitation. These were diarrhoea, enteritis and gastritis(2). Taken together they accounted for more than a third of infant deaths in a bad year. Children between the ages of three and nine months were particularly prone. Indeed, the World Health Organisation feels that it is unhelpful to differentiate diarrhoeal infections, and that a single category is sufficient(3). Their bacteriological investigations in underdeveloped countries failed to isolate a specific enteric pathogen (an organism exclusively producing diarrhoeal disease). However, they list several which are most often found in abnormal numbers in the intestinal tracts of diarrhoea patients, of which Shigella (the dysentry bacilli) are the most frequent(4). This represents little progress on the state of advanced knowledge at the turn of the century. At the end of last century, the German Escherich and an American called Booker identified a plethora of organisms, normally found in small numbers in the intestinal tract as the cause of infantile diarrhoea, whilst in the early twentieth century Flexner was able to isolate the bacillus dysenteriae in the stools of infant diarrhoea sufferers(5).

Clinical observations suggest, as one might expect, that there were rather more symptoms in connection with enteric infections than the presence of diarrhoea itself. Writing in 1893, Dr. Park, the medical officer of health for Houghton, stressed that, 'Young and old alike were affected' by diarrhoea and that the illness was 'characterized by cramps in the body and legs, vomiting and great prostration', as well as the obvious symptom(6). Park's observations are consistent with the course of the disease, which falls into three stages. Firstly, there is a fluid loss, accompanied by vomiting and nausea. The shock to the system which this causes explains the prostration noted by Park. Secondly, due to dehydration, a renal insufficiency may occur. This is unlikely in adults who will compensate easily by drinking liquids but the loss is likely to be much more serious in infancy. Depending on the extent of dehydration and on the treatment administered, if any, the third stage will either be convalescence and recovery, or death(7). The World Health Organisation considers that where the infant mortality rate is above 100 diarrhoea is endemic. Late nineteenth century Britain, or more specifically its urban areas, is clearly in this category(8). The fact that contemporaries, especially medical officers, did not make constant reference to stomach complaints is probably due to their acceptance as inevitable events. In particular, they were an inconvenience of the summer months, because although diarrhoea was endemic, it was also seasonal. Its visitations were generally restricted to the third quarter of the year when it often reached epidemic proportions. This produced a peak in general infant mortality in the third quarter, particularly during very hot summers.

The extent of the problem

Total infant mortality and infant diarrhoea
mortality rates in a number of colliery areas are
set out in Table 8.1. The infant mortality rate
has not been shown when diarrhoea mortality cannot
be differentiated. The data which are available
suggests that there was not a universal relationship between infant diarrhoea and general infant
mortality. Infant diarrhoea mortality was neither
a fixed proportion of total infant mortality, nor
was the rate of infant mortality, from all causes
other than diarrhoea, constant. Nevertheless,
years of excessive infant death were usually, though
not invariably, years when diarrhoea became
epidemic. There was a tendency for the infant
mortality rate to fluctuate with the level of
mortality from enteric infections. Diarrhoea
mortality did not account for the total fluctuation
but there appear to have been levels of infant
mortality which were not attained in years when
diarrhoea mortality was low. This is apparent
in Table 8.1 where, by and large, when the infant
mortality rate was 150, or more, the diarrhoea
rate was in excess of 30.
Unfortunately, the coverage in Table 8.1 is
less than comprehensive. It excludes the Durham
areas and it is almost totally confined to years
after 1900. This is not sufficient for a detailed
analysis. However, because the vast majority of
all diarrhoea deaths occurred in infancy, total
diarrhoea deaths (i.e. at all ages) per thousand
live births has been used as a substitute for infant
diarrhoea mortality. These are set out in Table
8.2.
Towards the end of last century medical
practitioners employed synonyms for diarrhoea to
an increasing extent. The principal ones were
enteritis and gastro-enteritis. This created problems because, at the time, they were differentiated
from diarrhoea in the classification of causes
of death used by the Registrar General of England
and Wales(9). This means that the diarrhoea mortality rates shown in Table 8.2 increasingly underestimate the true mortality from that cause. In
England and Wales by 1901 only two-thirds of infant
diarrhoea deaths were actually registered from
diarrhoea(10). This increasing tendency to underestimate should be borne in mind when Table 8.2
is examined. By and large, Table 8.1 conforms
to the pattern which is evident in Table 8.2. The

overall trend in diarrhoea was upwards towards the end of last century, although this tended to reverse as general infant mortality declined after 1900. Nevertheless diarrhoea continued to be a great source of danger to infants in epidemic years right up to the First World War. The level of diarrhoea mortality in 1911 demonstrates this. During the 1890s, the Glamorgan districts experienced a particularly large increase. It is possible that this was not a real change, but a product of changes in nomenclature on death certificates. Only deaths from convulsions could possibly have been interchangeable with diarrhoea on a scale sufficient to bring about an appreciable change in certified diarrhoea mortality rates. However, the diarrhoea death rates in the Glamorgan districts in the eighties appear to have been genuinely low because the infant mortality rate did not peak in the third quarter of the year. Infant mortality was usually at a maximum in the third quarter of the year in the Lancashire and Durham mining areas and in Lancashire Registration County, which was renowned as the principal diarrhoea county in England. However, Aberdare and Rhondda did not display diarrhoeal seasonality until 1892.

Infant feeding

Infant feeding is essentially a simple matter. Nature has provided mothers with a near perfect source of food for their children. A source, moreover, which is constantly at the right temperature and requires no preparation. Problems only arise when breast feeding is discontinued prematurely, either when the mother chooses to feed artificially, or loses the ability to feed naturally. The vulnerability of artificially or handfed infants meant that the promotion of breast feeding was a major platform in the early infant welfare movement(11). Propagandists illustrated the importance of breast feeding with the experience of the Lancashire cotton famine and the seige of Paris(12). Apparently, voluntary hand feeding in Paris and among cotton operatives was on such a scale that when normal life was disrupted and circumstances compelled mothers to feed at the breast the infant mortality rates fell despite the general hardship. The advent of health visitors in England and Wales made possible empirical demonstrations of these alleged advantages. Their records in the selected areas

Table 8.1: Mortality from infant diarrhoea

	Total Infant Mortality	Infant Diarrhoea Mortality	Non Diarrhoea Infant Mortality
RHONDDA U.D.			
1898	192.2	43.4	148.8
1899	244.1	80.7	163.4
1900	187.7	31.3	156.4
1901	222.4	58.2	164.2
1902	178.9	17.2	161.7
1903	-	-	-
1904	190.3	49.4	140.9
1905	206.3	40.8	165.5
1906	174.3	47.1	127.2
1907	161.9	25.5	136.4
1908	183.7	49.7	134.0
1909	-	-	-
1910	136.8	26.7	110.1
1911	164.3	59.6	104.7
INCE U.D.			
1902	190.3	61.9	128.4
1903	180.5	56.5	124.0
1904	226.3	95.6	130.7
1905	202.8	78.6	124.2
1906	181.6	65.9	115.7
1907	179.7	48.8	130.9
1908	183.3	42.9	140.4
1909	212.0	63.6	148.4
1910	165.1	33.8	131.3
ABERDARE U.D.			
1907	134.9	21.2	113.7
1908	212.7	38.8	173.9
1909	-	-	-
1910	151.2	30.5	120.7

Table 8.1: Continued

	Total Infant Mortality	Infant Diarrhoea Mortality	Non Diarrhoea Infant Mortality
WIGAN C.B.			
1902	164.0	18.6	145.4
1903	175.0	24.3	150.7
1904	188.0	34.6	153.4
1905	163.1	45.9	117.2
1906	160.3	38.7	121.6
1907	163.5	26.8	136.7
1908	154.4	37.2	117.2
1909	169.9	30.4	139.5
1910	132.9	21.7	111.2
1911	193.8	64.3	129.5
HINDLEY U.D.			
1905	151.1	47.1	100.3
1906	159.8	51.2	108.6
1907	152.2	34.7	117.5
1908	158.2	19.9	138.3
1909	176.1	22.0	154.1
1910	122.6	9.6	113.0
1911	146.5	35.2	111.3

Note: All rates calculated per thousand live births.

Source: Annual Reports of the Medical Officers of
Health for Rhondda U.D., Aberdare U.D.,
Wigan C.B., Ince U.D. and Hindley U.D.

Table 8.2: Deaths per Thousand live births, from Diarrhoea at all ages in selected Registration Areas

	Wigan	Hindley	Rhondda	Aberdare	Hetton	Houghton	England and Wales
1880-4	33.4	37.4	13.8	1.6	34.4	43.4	16.2
1885-9	30.0	28.4	9.8	7.8	28.8	33.6	15.2
1890-4	35.4	30.6	12.6	13.4	18.4	29.8	16.8
1895-9	31.6	35.8	30.8	39.4	13.6	39.2	31.4
1900-4	43.0	35.0	28.4	28.2	12.4	15.6	24.6
1905-9	30.4	41.4	35.4	16.4	21.6	15.4	19.6
1910	26.0	26.0	22.0	10.0	16.0	9.0	13.0
1899	37.0	40.0	46.0	75.0	19.0	21.0	40.0
1911 (a)	73.0	59.0	63.0	74.0	96.0	47.0	36.0

Note: (a) Calculated from deaths up to two years only.

Source: Quarterly Returns of the Registrar General for England and Wales, 1880-1911.

give an indication of the proportions of children fed naturally and by hand. Table 8.3 sets out the experience in some mining areas.

No records have been located for Houghton and Hetton but feeding practices seem to have been reasonably uniform in the other areas. Table 8.3 appears to suggest that hand fed infants ran the greatest risk of death, particularly from diarrhoea. In excess of two-thirds of all infants were wholly breast fed, whereas, in general, under one third of those dying of diarrhoea were totally breast fed. The figures do not control for the age at death of infant fatalities or age at inspection of survivors. Nevertheless, at a time when it was normal to lactate right through the first year the differences apparent in Table 8.3 remain significant. It also seems likely that there was a high level of breast feeding, though this is based on the experience in Rhondda alone.

The susceptibility of artificially fed infants to diarrhoea raises the question of whether breast feeding was declining during the period. Before the fall in the infant mortality rate in England and Wales, and in the colliery areas, perceptible rises took place in the 1890s. The importance of diarrhoeal deaths in these years led many contemporaries to blame the increase in infant mortality on artificial feeding. However, the extent of breast feeding during the first year after birth was not systematically recorded until the twentieth century. This means that changes in the pattern of infant feeding can only be surmised from other evidence, mainly concerned with motives and opportunities.

Economically there was little incentive to a non-earning mother to feed artificially because she had a free source of food at her disposal. If, as in the coalfields, employment was not an opportunity cost and the mother was healthy there was no pecuniary advantage to be gained by hand feeding. This consideration, coupled with their observations, led some experienced medical men to believe that inability to lactate forced artificial feeding on many mothers. It is important to remember that at the time it was quite common to breast feed until and even beyond the first birthday. Even allowing for some early voluntary weaning, loss of milk seems likely to have been a major consideration. The same point was put forcibly before the Inter-Departmental Committee on Physical Deterioration by Dr. Hutchison. He

Table 8.3: <u>Methods of feeding infants in the Select-</u>
<u>ed areas</u>

A. Data relating to all infants

Area	Breast fed (%)	Partially Breast fed (%)	Artifically fed (%)
Rhondda U.D.			
1910	68.5	12.1	19.5
1911	75.1	3.2	21.7

B. Data relating to infants dying from all causes

Rhondda U.D.			
1910	37.2	19.0	43.8
1911	30.5	10.7	58.8
Wigan C.B.			
1914	34.0	14.7	51.3

C. Data relating to infants dying from diarrhoea

Wigan C.B.			
1905	34.8	9.1	56.1
1906	23.0	4.3	72.7
1907	33.3	1.7	65.0
1908	21.8	2.3	75.9
1909	13.7	5.9	80.4
1910	9.8	9.8	80.4
1911	22.4	2.2	75.4
Ince U.D.			
1905	20.7	6.9	72.4
Rhondda U.D.			
1899	15.0	-	-
Aberdare U.D.			
1907	12.5	8.3	79.2

<u>Source</u>: Annual Reports of the Medical officers of
health for Rhondda U.D., Wigan C.B., Ince
U.D., and Aberdare U.D.

placed it on record that, 'it is a great pity; but it (premature weaning) is not a question of "will not" but "cannot". It would be unfair to say that the average mother at present refuses to suckle her own child; she is unable to do so in quite a large number of cases'(13). It is not difficult to enumerate problems in a working man's, particularly a miner's, way of life which placed stress on his wife and could have contributed to her ceasing to lactate. The sheer size of families exhausted many mothers and the shift system, with its varying hours for husbands and perhaps sons and lodgers, who were unable to wash and change at work, placed a heavy additional burden on colliers' wives. Moreover, despite relatively high wages a collier's wife was not necessarily well nourished. Wages were often dissipated and, even when they were not, it seems likely that the bread winner claimed the lion's share of the household diet.

If one accepts that involuntary cessation of breast feeding was the main cause of early weaning during the first part of this century, then one must assume that there had been little increase in artificial feeding over the last half of the nineteenth century. There is no reason to believe that the quality of life of working class mothers, including miners' wives, had fallen appreciably at that time. Indeed, rising real wages, ought, if anything, to have enhanced their material lives. Nevertheless, there were changes in the kinds of artificial infant feeds which were on the market. Alternatives to cows' milk appeared, particularly tinned condensed milk. It is conceivable that new substitutes for breast milk were less suitable than might have been thought at the time.

During the period in question there were three main alternatives to a mother's natural food; cows' milk, tinned condensed milk and patent/adults' food. Cows' milk was generally raw (untreated) since pasteurization was not common before the Great War. Milk depots and clinics often provided treated milk but this was usually sterilized rather than pasteurized. Condensed milk was of varied quality but the sweetened skimmed varieties were the cheapest and least suitable for babies. Patent foods and adult food have been grouped together because both were starchy and difficult for an infant to digest. It is impossible to gauge the extent to which infants were fed on morsels from their parents' plates but there is little to suggest that patent foods were widely used in the selected areas and there were variations in the extent to which different artificial foods were used in the selected areas.

It is interesting to notice that dried milk was never mentioned as a substitute feed. In the twentieth century it has become the accepted alternative to natural milk because exact quantities can be prepared, because the cleanliness of the source is certain, and because it is supplied in a form which may be stored safely. Despite the attempts of the Glaxo company to penetrate the British market, which included a full front page advertisement in the Daily Mail, it was 1911 before they had any success(14), and dried milk did not prove its worth to the majority of consumers until large numbers of mothers encountered it during World War I(15). As can be seen in the selected areas, prior to the acceptance of dried milk feeds condensed milk vied with cows' milk as the main substitute(16). This was particularly the case among the working classes, but there is no reason to believe that this represented any progress(17). Indeed the contrary seems to have been true. Most condensed milks were sweet and had to be diluted. Cheaper brands were made from skimmed milk and were short on milk fats which were essential for healthy development. The most apparent advantage of condensed milk, its purity, was irrelevent in working class homes. Tins were opened and left exposed to the risks of pollution, especially by flies. Tin openers were not a universally owned utensil; and there is evidence that shopkeepers opened tins for customers(18). This was dangerous because the sugar in condensed milk attracted flies, and they carried disease. Newsholme was particularly aware of the dangers presented to infant life by the combination of flies and condensed milk(19):

> The sugar used in sweetening milk is often black with flies, which may have come from a neighbouring dustbin or manure heap, or from the liquid stools of a diarrhoeal patient in a neighbouring house. Flies have to be picked out of the half empty can of condensed milk before its remaining contents can be used for the next meal.

This was a problem which was exacerbated by inadequate food storage facilities like those described in Houghton: 'In the workmens' cottages

the pantries are often small and badly ventilated
so that in the summer months the food rapidly
decomposes and has a very hurtful effect especially
on the young'(20).

All artificial foods became more dangerous
if they were carelessly dispensed, and from the
end of the nineteenth century there was considerable
debate over the merits of different types of feeding
bottles. The medical officers for both Rhondda
and Aberdare were struck by the prevalence of the
long-tube feeding bottle, which was difficult to
clean between feeds. In the Rhondda in 1899 only
two cases of the more satisfactory boat bottle
(basically that still in use to-day) were recorded
amongst the diarrhoea fatalities, whilst in 1910
72 per cent of all bottles used were of the long-
tube type(21). Dr. Spencer Low noted, in his report
on Aberdare in 1907, that he 'saw a very large
number of artificially fed babies during the course
of (his) inspection, and long-tube feeding bottles
were in common use. Very rarely indeed the more
satisfactory boat shaped bottle was seen'(22).
These were unfortunate observations because the
long india-rubber tube which made feeding easy
because of its flexibility, could not be adequately
cleaned and traces of previous feeds remained to
attract flies or turn sour.

On balance the evidence suggests that hand
feeding did not increase significantly at the end
of the nineteenth century, but there was a relationship between the method of feeding and diarrhoea
mortality. Artificially-fed infants were more
likely to die from an enteric infection than breast-
fed infants. Furthermore, a Local Government Board
investigation demonstrated that infants fed on
condensed milk were more likely to die of diarrhoea
than infants fed on raw cows' milk. The chances
of death from diarrhoea were about twice as great
among infants fed on condensed milk(23). Thus
the increasing use of condensed milk, albeit only
at the expense of raw cows' milk, assumes importance
in the context of the rising diarrhoea mortality
in the 1890s. The use of condensed milk must,
in itself, have contributed to this mortality.
However, the extent of any contribution is difficult to measure because the whole question was
further complicated by the occurrence of a series
of good summers at the end of the nineteenth cen-
tury(24). The influence of hot weather on enteric
infections has already been noted. The poor summers
of the 1880s and the early 1890s, followed by the

better weather thereafter, culminating in the heatwave in 1899, pushed up diarrhoeal deaths. This
made the effects of artificial feeding more evident
but obscured the impact of condensed milk. Before
any overall evaluation of diarrhoeal mortality
can be attempted, the significance of summer weather
and sanitary provision must be considered.

Musca domestica

A great deal has been made of the relationship
between breast feeding and diarrhoea. However,
the middle and upper classes more often had recourse
to artificial food than the working classes, yet
their infant diarrhoea and general infant mortality
rates were lower(25). This paradox is resolved
when one realises that artificial feeding did not
itself cause diarrhoea but that its significance
was that it made infection easier. The higher
standards of cleanliness of the middle and upper
classes, both environmental and personal, prevented
artificial feeding from producing heavy diarrhoea
mortality. It was poor sanitation and hygiene
together with artificial feeding which brought
diarrhoea. A variety of vectors, that is agencies
transmitting the bacteria, were involved in the
infective process. However, one vector in particular was important because it gave the bacteria
the power to fly and it was consistent with the
detailed observations of contemporaries, and with
the pattern of diarrhoea mortality in the mining
areas. That vector was the fly in its common
varieties and in particular the numerous house
fly (musca domestica). Although now everyday knowledge, the importance of flies as carriers
of disease was only suspected until the early
twentieth century because little was known about
their behaviour(26). An examination of the life
cycle and habits of musca domestica demonstrates
its importance in enteric infection and establishes
the main link between the environment and infant
feeding(27).
Musca domestica is not a pleasant creature.
The female lays between 100 and 150 eggs at a time,
in manure, refuse or other organic matter. These
hatch within twenty-four hours and the next stage
in the life cycle, the larval, lasts for about
a week. Prior to the pupal stage the larva buries
itself in the ground, and it is here that the pupa
forms and hatches into the adult fly in between
three and 25 days, according to the temperature

of its surroundings(28). House-flies pick up bacteria when feeding on or laying their eggs in faeces. They either adhere directly to the body or are taken up the proboscis with the digestive juices and enter the alimentary canal. On visiting human food, bacteria may be transferred directly from the creature's body or during regurgitation which is practised to liquify food for the fly's consumption(29). During the hot summer the earth temperature increases and musca domestica's life cycle can be shortened by as much as 22-25 days, to only 8-11 days. A shorter life cycle produces adult flies quicker, and they in turn breed in the same suitable conditions and produce a plague. The life cycle itself spreads infection to unsuspecting humans. This process is exacerbated when the weather is still and dry, as well as hot, because this increases musca domestica's mobility. The operation of the fly vector is in evidence in Rhondda, where the medical officer recorded weekly earth temperatures and weekly numbers of deaths from diarrhoea in the years after 1899. The pupa of the common house-fly incubates in the subsoil. This takes time to absorb the sun's heat sufficiently to retain warmth through the hours of darkness. Until this happens flies do not hatch in large numbers. The temperature of the earth at a few feet depth is an indicator of the build-up of heat in the subsoil. It was recorded in the Rhondda at a depth of four feet and tabulated in the medical officer's annual reports along with weekly diarrhoea mortality. It is evident that the week with the highest earth temperature general-ly was the week with the highest number of diarrhoea deaths, and that the vast majority of diarrhoea deaths always followed the attainment of the summer's maximum earth temperature. That is after the house-fly had reached its peak breeding period. Furthermore, fatalities were never high in June because the year's flies had not hatched, and had diarrhoea depended simply on the putrefaction of waste, or the souring of milk and the decay of food, one would have anticipated epidemics in June when the air temperature was often high. The autumn incidence of diarrhoea was a universal observation. All the data in the selected areas confirm this.

This primacy of the fly vector means that the factors combining to produce infant diarrhoea deaths were filth and artificial feeding. It was the method of disposing of excrement and other waste products rather than overcrowding and poor

housing which caused diarrhoea, although a lack
of washing facilities in an overcrowded home were
important because they lowered standards of personal
hygiene. An examination of the sanitary conditions
in the selected areas reveals a multitude of possible sources of infection.

Sewage and potable water

The disposal of human excreta was crucial
because it was a source of bacteria and a feeding
ground and resting place for flies. These might,
in turn, share human food with some unsuspecting
individual and spread infection. There are two
methods of dealing with human waste: immediate
removal by a water carriage system, which has become
universal in twentieth century Britain, and any
of a number of conservancy systems, which store
excreta for periodic removal. There are two main
types of conservancy system: that using a cess
pit or midden which is emptied infrequently, say
twice a year, and the pail or ash closet system
which has to be emptied regularly, at best daily.
On the basis that the system which most rapidly
removes excrement from in and around human habita-
tions is preferable, because it reduces sources
of bacterial infection, the water carriage system
is the most suitable. The persistence of diarrhoea
in the years before World War I is explicable at
a basic level because conservancy systems were
still widespread in Britain in these years(30).
However, without affecting this general explanation
the actuality was more complex. Although the
superiority of water closets is unquestioned several
constraints reduced the efficiency of water carriage
systems. Not all W.C.'s were fitted with water
boxes or cisterns. In some cases to economize
on water, waste water had to be poured directly
into the bowl. When this chore was neglected the
cleanliness of closets deteriorated and the advantage of a water carriage system was lost. Moreover,
general maintenance and cleaning were themselves
an independent problem, particularly when a W.C.
was shared by several households and no one took
responsibility for these essential tasks. Even
when each household had its own W.C., and this
was fitted with a cistern, the efficiency of the
system was impaired if at anytime the water supply
failed. A water carriage system without water
is no system at all. This danger was compounded
because droughts were most likely during the

diarrhoea epidemic season, at the end of hot
summers. Water was also needed to flush sewers
and prevent their stagnation. Interruptions in
supply also made it increasingly difficult to maintain standards of domestic cleanliness, particularly
when water was not piped into the house anyway(31).
The effectiveness of conservancy systems also
varied. The abdication of responsibility for the
cleanliness of shared closets was more damaging
in a conservancy system. When the excrement which
had accumulated in a midden had to be removed the
task was unpleasant. It was particularly unhealthy
in those cases where, in the absence of rear access,
it had to be carried through the houses. Where
pails were used they became hazards when, for any
reason, they were not scavenged. Their superiority
over pits and middens depended on regular removal.
Moreover, if general scavenging was interrupted,
refuse began to decompose and became a source of
infection and a breeding ground for flies. Even
when vigilance was maintained, the problem was
sometimes concentrated in particular parts of a
district because refuse and nightsoil were taken
to tips sited close to houses. All these problems
existed in mining areas.

The two Glamorgan areas established a water
carriage system for sewage disposal earlier than
the other districts. The Rhondda was sewered to
the sea, via Pontypridd, by 1893, at which time
over half of the houses (mainly in newer developments) had W.C.'s which had previously emptied
into the rivers. Plans for the main sewer to the
sea were ready by 1888 and work began in the following year, as plans for the Rhondda sewer were final-
ized. As these main arteries neared completion
it was decided that existing closets should be
converted to a water carriage system and that all
new provision should be W.C.'s(32). In 1897 4,290
houses were not connected to the sewer but by 1905
only 451 were without W.C.'s and only 158 were
without by 1912(33). This process was not without
problems, principally caused by subsidence which
dogged schemes in mining districts. Cracked and
broken pipes impaired the efficiency of sewers,
and inflated maintenance costs were often sufficient
to discourage the extension of the water carriage
system to many districts.

The vigilance of the medical officers from
Rhondda which provides invaluable evidence of sanitation and scavenging is equally informative about
the provision of water in the district. Throughout

the 1880s the water supply of the two major water
companies was inadequate. The Ystrad Gas and Water
Company which supplied the Rhondda Fawr down to
the Miskin Hotel, Trealaw and the Gethin Hotel,
Penygraig had insufficient storage space whilst
the Pontypridd water company which supplied the
rest of the district failed to meet its obligations
because its main reservoir leaked(34). As early
as 1880 a municipal take-over of the Ystrad Company
was mooted but no action was taken when assurances
were given that the service would be improved(35).
However, shortages persisted, domestic supplies
were discontinued and drains were not flushed,
until at the end of the decade the matter reached
a head. The Pontypridd Company had not remedied
their leak nor had the Ystrad Company built adequate
storage capacity and the medical officer reported
that 'the two chief water supplies of your district
were, during the summer months, very deficient
in quantity and of second class quality...(and)...
It is an open secret that filtration is
only occasionally practised by...(these)... water
companies'(36). The importance of the water supply
was impressed on the authorities by the impending
construction of the sewer to the sea and the increased demand which this would place on already
strained supplies. This fundamental inability
to meet the demand of the district was exacerbated
by the valleys' geography which made pumping stations necessary to counter the sharply changing
levels. Indeed there were many houses without
any supply in the nineties which made use of wells
and spouts (pistyllau) on the hillsides(37). Moreover, problems with the main companies were not
confined to shortages, the quality of the supply
often failed to come up to standard. The Pontypridd
Company was especially at fault on this count.
It was normal for the supply to become undrinkable
in the summer months because it contained a peaty
suspension(38). In 1890 two putrid frogs were
found in service pipes and sheep clippings were
found in the supply. The Ystrad Company was
suspected of drawing water from the river at a
point below the entry of waste from a small house
coal colliery. It is conceivable that this could
have been polluted by the workmen's excrement.
Nevertheless, when they brought an action, the
local authority could not obtain a conviction.
The medical officer was incensed and pointed to
more numerous deaths from diarrhoea in areas served
by the Pontypridd Company as evidence of its

inadequacy(39). In June 1891, during a visit to
the water works by the chamber of commerce, Mr.
Baynes, the works' manager, was asked how he got
such good chemical reports for his water and
answered: 'You see we have such a large volume
of pure water coming down here that a little filth
don't tell'(40).
    The institution of a water carriage system
came later in the Lancashire areas. The process
only really began in Wigan County Borough in 1896.
By 1898 there were 1,431 W.C.'s and 8,446 other
types of convenience, mainly pail closets(41).
By the time Pemberton Urban District was grafted
on to the old County Borough in 1905(42), Wigan
had about half as many W.C.'s as conservancy conveniences. Pemberton, however, was mainly provided
for by privy middens so the enlarged County Borough
had 1,669 middens, 7,849 pail closets and 6,900
W.C.'s in 1912(43). The subdistrict, which kept
the boundaries of the old County Borough of Wigan,
had improved and was almost free from middens by
that time. In the 1870s diarrhoea mortality had
been particularly excessive in Wigan and was only
moderated when large middens were replaced by pails
in which excreta was mixed with ashes and removed
regularly. At the same time a proper sewer was
laid and it became possible to advance, albeit
slowly, towards a water carriage system. Pails
with an ash mixture predominated until just before
World War I. They were regularly scavenged and
the contents were taken away in the pails which
were fitted with sprung lids. They were used as
manure on agricultural land, unless there was an
enteric fever outbreak in which case red tubs were
provided to the houses concerned. This was an
indication that the contents were to be incinerated.
As the water carriage system developed the sewage
was treated by irrigation on a sewage farm. In
the early years of this century this was located
at Hoscar Moss, half way to Southport. Wigan was
not exempt from the subsidence which was found
in Glamorgan. Indeed, in parts of Wigan, the Leeds
and Liverpool canal was above the level of the
surrounding land. Many drains and sewers dated
from 1852. By the early twentieth century these
were extensively fractured but it was claimed that
seepage was less than might have been thought
because the joints were made of a malleable clay
'puddle', rather than the more rigid cement(44).
Paradoxically, this was a practice which was criticized elsewhere. The medical officer testified

to the efficacy of the mid-nineteenth century reforms in his report to his employers in 1896: 'We
may safely say that since the old privy system
of excrement removal has been abolished, and the
sewerage system been attended to, that the diarrhoea
which used to be so prevalent 25 years ago has
disappeared, and this is through improved sanitation'(45). This was certainly the case but, by
standards other than its own recent history, Wigan
was still an area of excessive infant diarrhoea
mortality in the 1890s.

Whilst pails remained there were ample sources
of infection, although, ironically, the problem
was concentrated by increased efficiency in
scavenging. Flies bred in refuse: where improvement
had occurred, and long term conservancy had been
replaced by a system which involved regular removal
of excreta but stopped short of a universal water
carriage system, plagues of flies still caused
havoc. The solution lay in the provision of refuse
depots at a distance from housing and a completely
water carriage sewage system.

In 1886 it was reported that the Wigan water
supply was constant and good, an opinion which
was reiterated in 1894. The supply came from moor-
land at Hassock Hill after being filtered through
sand and gravel(46). However, it is clear that
a constant supply does not mean that there were
never shortages, since the medical officer reported
that the supply was intermittent and of uncertain
quality in the summer of 1896.

In Hindley sub-district (Abram, Hindley and
Ince Urban Districts) the position was similar
to that in Wigan County Borough. In the eighties
privy middens abounded and scavenging was unsatisfactory. At Ince privies were of an inadequate
type and in short supply, though improved forms
were being introduced. Scavenging was also
inadequate and yards were frequently unpaved and
filthy with excrement slops and other refuse. In
Abram unsatisfactory scavenging was found in
combination with 'deep, wet and offensive' midden
privies(47). The position in Hindley Urban District
was similar though there were already some pails
in use, but drains do not seem to have
been trapped(48). Over the next two decades
improvements were made. The most offensive middens
were removed but progress towards a water carriage
system was slow. In 1911 only about one closet
in five was a W.C. (21.7 per cent in Hindley,
22 per cent in Ince and 14.8 per cent in Abram),

and the conservancy system remained largely
a midden, rather than a pail, system(49). In 1911
Dr. Manby, making a Local Government Board inspection, felt able to report substantial improvement
in the cleanliness of Ince in the quarter of a
century since the previous inspection, but he
lamented that the town was still a privy midden
one(50). In Hindley Urban District 60 new W.C.'s
were constructed each year between 1907 and 1912;
and of these 91 were conversions; 8 in 1907, 5
in 1908, 15 in 1909, 5 in 1910 and 58 in 1911(51).
Improvement was belated and did not proceed at
breakneck speed. In Ince, midden privies remained
far more common than in Hindley Urban District
and this conbributed to the higher levels
of diarrhoea mortality in Ince during the first
decade of this century.

The sanitary background to Houghton and Hetton
was apparently worse than that in the Glamorgan
or Lancashire areas. In 1914 Hetton Urban District
had only 235 W.C.'s compared to 2,626 ash closets
and privies, whilst Houghton Urban District had
451 W.C.'s to 1,466 conservancy conveniences and
there were only 150 W.C.'s to 4,900 closets and
privies in the Rural District(52). Thus 23.5 per
cent of all closets were W.C.'s in Houghton Urban
District and only 8.2 per cent and 3 per cent in
Hetton Urban District and Houghton Rural District
respectively. The problem of primitive facilities
in the Durham areas was compounded by less than
satisfactory scavenging of middens. In the introduction to a report on a Local Government Board
inspection in County Durham, made in 1910, Newsholme
remarked that, 'The importance of careful and frequent scavenging may be gathered from the repulsive
details which it has been Dr. Wheaton's duty to
place on record'(53). A short passage from Wheaton
himself gives an indication of the filth abounding
in the worst parts of the County(54):

> Many of the privies are very large with un-
> covered receptacles sunk below the ground
> level, not water tight, and serving for two,
> four or a much larger number of houses. In
> some districts many of these privies are great-
> ly dilapidated and without proper doors, so
> that their contents escape on the surface
> of the streets...in which they are situated.

Moreover, by necessity they were close to housing.
Even in the less desperate areas poor scavenging

complicated the sanitary situation. In the early part of the period scavenging of closets was generally left to tenants. This created two main problems. Firstly, when responsibility was shared it was apt to be neglected. In 1884 the medical officer for Houghton Urban District reported that, 'The ashpits are emptied more regularly than formerly'. In the second place, because tenants would not pay to hire carts to remove excreta they had to rely on farmers collecting it for use as manure. Dr. Park pointed out, in 1883, that this meant that:(55)

> They...(were)...obliged to wait the convenience of the farmers who at certain seasons of the year...(were)...too much occupied with their farm work to be able to remove the ashes with any degree of regularity. And if it is true as many of...(the farmers)...aver that the ashes are hardly worth the carting away this is not to be wondered at when it is remembered that they get nothing for their trouble.

Farmers were, of course, busiest at harvest time which coincided with autumn diarrhoea. Responsibility fell increasingly on landlords but still the problem persisted because tenders were accepted from local men with carts and, of course, most of the carts in the district were owned by the self same farmers who had previously scavenged for nothing.

The water supply for the Durham districts came from diverse sources. The supply for Houghton Urban District came from the shaft of Houghton pit at a depth of forty fathoms. The Northern Division of the Rural District relied on three main sources, the Grass Well, the Boiling Well, the Newbottle and Penshaw Water Company. Some outlying districts took their supplies from local springs(56). In Hetton and the Southern Division supplies were equally varied. Hetton's supply came from the same source as the Sunderland and South Shields Water Company, West Rainton was supplied by the Durham and Shildon Water Company, and the Shildon and Waskerly Water Company and the Weardale Water Company were also involved in the district. The Weardale Water Company was criticized for supplying outlying districts by barrel as late as 1896(57). Early reports all claimed that supplies were abundant and clean but

as standards rose, and significance was attached
to shortages, medical officers began to report
them. Springs were particularly susceptable in
summer months and, as in other areas, main supplies
were also vulnerable. In Houghton Urban District
water supplies were discontinued after 11 p.m.
during the summer of 1898 and the following year
shortages were again reported. In Hetton, the
Middle Rainton supply was sometimes irregular and
springs were fickle in Moorsley and East Rain-
ton(58). Intermittent supplies in Hetton were
recorded by the County Medical Officer in 1901
and 1903 , and in Houghton Urban District between
1904 and 1907(59).

In Houghton and Hetton there were greater
problems over the purity of the supply than elsewhere. In 1882 the Local Government Board's reports
contain an account of an outbreak of enteric fever
in New Herrington which originated in the water
supply. This became contaminated by human excrement which was thrown down a fissure at a nearby
farm(60). Concern over quality became general
in the nineties with the institution of systematic
chemical analyses of supplies. The supply in
Houghton Urban District was of doubtful quality
in the early nineties, at which time a search began
for alternative supplies. In the northern division
contamination of the Herrington supply caused concern even after the typhoid epidemic(61). Both
of these supplies were subject to intermittent
pollution, 'not connected with disease' (sic),
right up to 1900(62).

Conclusion

The accumulated experience in the selected
areas suggests that bacteria found in urban filth,
carried by flies to artificially fed infants, was
the main method of transmitting diarrhoeal disease.
The potential of flies as a vector in enteric
infections can be established with reference to
the life cycle of the common house-fly. Its breeding and feeding habits link it with excreta, which
are the bacterial source, and infant food. However,
it is the coincidence of the peak breeding period
of flies and of infant diarrhoea, in the autumn
of each year, which suggests that the house-fly
was an important element in the infective process.
The series of weekly earth temperatures, which
determined when house-flies hatched, and weekly
diarrhoea mortality in Rhondda strongly support

this hypothesis.

There is little evidence that hand feeding of infants increased as infant mortality increased in the 1890s. Nor can this temporary increase in diarrhoea mortality be explained by a deterioration in sanitary provision. The explanation lies in the run of fine summers at the end of the century, which led up to the 1899 heatwave. These were favourable to the breeding of flies. Additionally, although the amount of artificial feeding did not increase, condensed milk was increasing in popularity as an infant feed. The sugar, which most brands of condensed milk contained, attracted flies more than raw cows' milk. This meant that infants who were fed on condensed milk were the most vulnerable to enteric infection, and that its increasing popularity exacerbated the effects of the hot summers.

The sanitary provisions, the systems of refuse removal and the water supplies in all the selected areas provided many sources of infection and breeding grounds for flies. Mining villages and towns were notoriously insanitary places. What is interesting, however, is how different aspects of the environment assumed importance in diarrhoea infection in the various selected areas. In the Glamorgan areas there were water carriage sewage systems. The water carriage system is associated with the rapid and effective removal of sewage. However, the system broke down in Aberdare and Rhondda, primarily because the water supply failed regularly during the autumn months of the year. A water carriage system without water is worse than a conservancy system. In the Lancashire districts, the problem lay in the continued dependence on a conservancy system. Water carriage systems were being introduced in both areas but middens and pails remained the main method of sewage removal up to the Great War. Ironically, as the experience in Wigan demonstrates, the substitution of regularly scavenged pails for middens was a mixed blessing because it concentrated the source of infection around the refuse depots. Wigan was an urban area, and as in Rhondda and Aberdare, refuse was dumped in close proximity to houses. Nevertheless, infant diarrhoea mortality was, in general, greatest in the Ince area of Hindley where middens were common. In the Durham areas, the major problems were the breakdown of scavenging in the diarrhoeal months, and the use of a conservancy system. Houghton and Hetton were largely

rural and depended on farmers to scavenge pails
and middens. Unfortunately, farmers were busy
with harvest when the need to scavenge most scrup-
ulously was greatest.
By and large, conservancy sewage disposal,
particularly the midden variety, presented the
greatest source of enteric infection. The difficulties experienced with water carriage in
Glamorgan were exceptions, albeit interesting and
important ones. In the Durham areas sanitary
provision was as bad as anywhere, including Ince,
and yet, in general, diarrhoea mortality was not
excessive, though in epidemic years it was extremely
high(63). This demonstrates the potential for
infection which existed. The failure of enteric
infections to claim an annual proportion of deaths
consistent with the viscousness of the environment
was a function of the rural nature of the mining
industry in that county. Houghton and Hetton were
made up of scattered communities. Filth abounded
but it was not concentrated as it was in Wigan
or Ince, or by the steep valley sides in Glamorgan.
The close proximity of dense populations and filth
brings together bacterial sources, breeding grounds
for flies and maximum opportunities for them to
contaminate infant foods. The distinction involved
here was drawn succinctly by G.D.H. Cole: 'Twelve
insanitary houses on a hillside may be a picturesque
village, but twelve hundred are a grave nuisance,
and twelve thousand a pest and a horror'(64).
Over the period 1880-1911, and particularly
after 1900, steady improvements were made in the
sanitary provision and water supplies in all districts, although they were limited in Houghton
and Hetton. Despite this the position never became
satisfactory before World War I. The very hot
summer of 1911 brought a return of excessive infant
diarrhoea mortality in the autumn. This illustrated
that many inadequacies remained. In the inter-
war years water carriage sewage systems were
extended and continuous water supplies ensured,
and, together with other changes, the introduction
of dried milk feeds and maternity clinics suggesting
themselves as the most important, this helped to
dramatically reduce infant diarrhoea mortality.
A broad spectrum of reforms and changes in child
handling practice were necessary before the favourable position vis-a-vis infant diarrhoea, which
we enjoy today, was reached. This article has
pursued the question on a singular basis, that
of bacterial infection via a fly vector, because

171

this is the most plausible line of research in the conditions which prevailed around the turn of the century. This does not mean that there was only one infective process. The environment was sufficiently bad in the selected areas for many to suggest themselves, and there was a contemporary lobby which felt, with some justification, that milk was contaminated on farms and delivered having already been infected(65). The contention is that the fly was of central importance as a vector because of the coherence it gives to the seasonal pattern of infant diarrhoea mortality.

NOTES

1. These six areas were registration sub-districts. They have been chosen, along with two others, to provide local case studies in a larger piece of research into infant mortality in British coal mining communities, between 1880 and 1911. One of the criteria which were used to select the areas requires some amplification here, so that sources can be checked and ambiguities in the text can be avoided. In order to maximize data sources, registration sub-districts were chosen because they corresponded, either exactly or closely, with sanitary areas. This means that the experience of local registrars and medical officers of health can be brought to bear on the question. The correspondences are as follows:

Registration sub-districts	Sanitary areas
Aberdare	Aberdare Urban District (U.D.)
Rhondda	Rhondda U.D.
Wigan	Wigan County Borough (C.B.)
Hindley	(Abram U.D., and (Hindley U.D., and (Ince in Makerfield U.D. (taken together.
Houghton	Houghton U.D. and the northern division of Houghton Rural District (R.D.)
Hetton	The southern division of Houghton R.D. and, from 1985, Hetton U.D. (the

Registration sub-   Sanitary areas
districts

                     total area remaining
                     unchanged throughout).

Until 1897 Rhondda U.D. was known as
Ystradyfodwg U.D. and until 1911 Rhondda sub-
district was known as Ystradyfodwy sub-district. However, to maintain continuity,
Rhondda has been used throughout in the text,
but not in notes.

2. These headings cover gastro-enteritis and
    a number of less important causes e.g. gastro-
    intestinal catarrh.
3. World Health Organisation, Technical Report
    Series No. 288, Enteric Infections (Geneva,
    1964), pp. 5-6.
4. Ibid. pp. 8-9.
5. B. Kramer and A. Kanof, 'Diarrhoea in Children:
    a Historical Review', Journal of Paediatrics,
    LVII (1960), p. 773.
6. Houghton le Spring Urban District, Annual
    Report of the Medical Officer of Health (1893).
7. World Health Organisation, op.cit. p.14 and
    G. Newman, Infant Mortality: A Social Problem
    (1906), p. 140.
8. World Health Organisation, op.cit. p.4.
9. 63rd Annual Report of the Registrar General
    for England and Wales for 1901 Parliamentary
    Papers, 1902, XVIII, p.li.
10. Ibid.
11. G.F. McCleary, The Maternity and Child Welfare
    Movement (1935).
12. W.O. Henderson, The Lancashire Cotton Famine,
    1861-5 (New York, 1969), pp. 104-5. See for
    example H.T. Ashby, Infant Mortality (Cam-
    bridge, 1915), p. 46.
13. Report of the Inter-Departmental Committee
    on Physical Deterioration Parliamentary Papers,
    1904, XXXII, Q.9909.
14. Sir Harry Jephcott, The First Fifty Years
    (1969), pp. 77-81.
15. In the selected areas see County of Durham,
    Quarterly Report of the Superintendent Health
    Visitor (Sept. 1915), and County of Lancaster,
    Report of the Public Health and Housing Com-
    mittee (Jan. 1919).
16. Condensed milk was popularly known as 'Swiss
    milk' because of the importance of the Swiss
    based Nestle's company as suppliers. The

steady growth of retained imports of condensed milk during the nineties and the Edwardian period is some indication of its growing popularity; see D.J. Oddy, 'The Working Class Diet, 1886-1914' (Unpublished Ph.D. thesis, University of London, 1971), p. 151.

17. c.f. M.W. Beaver, 'Infant Mortality and Milk', Population Studies, XXVIII, (1973), p. 244.

18. J. Blackman, 'Child Health and Diet in the Nineteenth Century', Society for the Social History of Medicine Bulletin, XIII (1974), p. 12.

19. Local Government Board, Further Preliminary Reports on Flies as Carriers of Infection, Report on Public Health and Medical Matters No. 16, (1909), p. 21.

20. Houghton le Spring Rural District (northern division), Annual Report of the Medical Officer of Health (1899).

21. Rhondda U.D., A.R. of the M.O.H. (1899), p. 47; (1910), p. 19.

22. Local Government Board, Report on the Sanitary Circumstances of Aberdare U.D. by Dr. J. Spencer Low (1907), p. 14.

23. Local Government Board, Report of an Enquiry into Condensed Milks; with special reference to their use as infant foods, Report on Public Health and Medical Matters No. 56, (1911), pp. 38-9.

24. 74th A.R. of the R.G. for England and Wales (1911), Parliamentary Papers 1912-3, XIII, Table XXII, p. xxxiv.

25. Ibid. Table 28b.

26. The Local Government Board investigated the role of flies as carriers of disease at this time. See Reports on Public Health and Medical Matters (New Series), Nos. 5, 16, 40, 53, 66, 85, and 102.

27. It should be emphasized that it is not maintained that flies were the only link between the environment and infant feeds, nor is it maintained that all diarrhoeas were infectious.

28. K.R. Snow, Insects and Disease (1974), p.61.

29. Ibid. p. 62.

30. 42nd Annual Report of the Local Government Board, Parliamentary Papers, 1913, XXXI, Appendix I, No. 39.

31. Supply by standpipe was the rule rather than the exception during the period.

32. Ystradyfodwg U.D., A.R. of the M.O.H. (1888),

p. 10; (1889), p. 11; and (1891), p. 10.

33. Rhondda U.D., A.R. of the M.O.H. (1905), p.44
    and Supplement to the 42nd Annual Report of
    the Medical Officer to the Local Government
    Board containing A Second Report on Infant
    and Child Mortality Parliamentary Papers,
    1913, XXXIII, p. 306.
34. Ystradyfodwg U.D., A.R. of the M.O.H. (1893),
    pp. 22-23.
35. Ibid. (1880), p. iv.
36. Ibid. (1889), p. 10.
37. Ibid. (1893), p. 23.   There were several other
    supplies besides the two main companies, see
    Ibid. (1889), p. 10.   Moreover, the position
    in the early nineties was the product of much
    recent improvement: 'Even as late as 1880...
    (only 44 per cent of houses in the Rhondda
    valleys)...received piped water.'   See E.D.
    Lewis, The Rhondda Valleys: A Study in Indust-
    rial Development (1959), p. 205.
38. Ystradyfodwg U.D., A.R. of the M.O.H. (1890),
    p. 11; (1891), p. 11; and Rhondda U.D., A.R.
    of the M.O.H. (1900), p. 92.
39. Ystradyfodwg U.D., A.R. of the M.O.H. (1890),
    pp. 11-12.
40. Ibid. (1891), p. 10.
41. W. Berry, 'Sanitary Progress in Wigan During
    the Last 30 Years', The Scalpel, (1898), re-
    print of his presidential address to the Wigan
    Medical Society.
42. Until 1904 Wigan County Borough and Wigan
    registration sub-district were coterminus.
    Thereafter the County Borough was enlarged
    by the addition of Pemberton U.D. and the
    sub-district retained its existing boundaries.
43. Local Government Board, Report on the General
    Sanitary Circumstances and Administration
    of the County Borough of Wigan, with Special
    Reference to Infant Mortality, by Dr. Monckton
    Copeman (1907), p. 7.; and Wigan C.B., A.R.
    of the M.O.H. (1912).
44. Local Government Board, op.cit. (Monckton
    Copeman 1907), p. 2. and pp. 6-8.
45. Wigan C.B., A.R. of the M.O.H. (1896), p.
    24.
46. Supplement to the 16th Annual Report of the
    Local Government Board Containing the Report
    of the Medical Officer for 1886. Parliamentary
    Papers, 1887, XXXVI, Appendix 10(a), Abstract
    of Inspectors' Reports on the Sanitary Survey,
    pp. 158-9 and Supp. to the 24th A.R. of the

L.G.B. containing the Report of the M.O. for 1894-5, Parliamentary Papers, 1896, XXXVII, The Inland Sanitary Survey, p. 245.

47. Supp. to the 16th A.R. of the L.G.B. containing the Report of the M.O. (1886), Parliamentary Papers, 1887, XXXVI, App. 10(a), p. 159.

48. Ibid. App. 12, Abstracts of Medical Inspections, p. 292.

49. 42nd A.R. of the L.B.G. Parliamentary Papers, 1913, XXXI, Appendix I, No. 39, pp. 196-8.

50. Supp. to the 40th A.R. of the L.G.B. containing the Report of the M.O. (1911-12), Parliamentary Papers, 1912-13, XXXVI, App. A No. 6, Abstracts of Medical Inspections, p. 154.

51. 42nd A.R. of the L.G.B. Parliamentary Papers, 1913, XXXI, Appendix I, No. 39, p. 196.

52. County of Durham, Annual Report of the Medical Officer of Health (1914).

53. Local Government Board, Preliminary Report on Enteric Fever in the County of Durham by Dr. S.W. Wheaton (1910), p. 4.

54. Ibid.

55. Houghton U.D., A.R. of the M.O.H. (1884); (1883), p. 6.

56. Supp. to the 24th A.R. of the L.G.B. containing the Report of the M.O. (1894-5), Parliamentary Papers, 1896, XXXVII, The Inland Sanitary Survey, p. 108; and Houghton R.D. (northern division), A.R. of the M.O.H. (1891).

57. Hetton U.D., A.R. of the M.O.H. (1898), and Houghton R.D. (southern division), A.R. of the M.O.H. (1889), (1896), pp. 5-6 and (1899), p. 6.

58. Houghton U.D., A.R. of the M.O.H. (1898), p. 6 and (1899), p. 5; and Houghton R.D., (southern division), A.R. of the M.O.H. (1885), p. 10.

59. County of Durham, A.R. of the M.O.H. (1901), p. 61; (1903), p. 49; (1904), p. 42; (1906), p. 40 and (1907), p. 46.

60. Local Government Board, Report of a Medical Inspection of the Northern Division of Houghton le Spring Rural District by Dr. Page (1889), pp. 2-7.

61. Houghton U.D., A.R. of the M.O.H. (1891); and Houghton R.D. (northern division), A.R. of the M.O.H. (1897), p. 14.

62. Houghton U.D., A.R. of the M.O.H. (1892), (1893), and (1895); and Houghton R.D. (northern division), A.R. of the M.O.H. (1896), and (1897), p. 14.

63. See Table 8.2, particularly the period 1895-9 and the individual years 1899 and 1911. These cover the main epidemic years.
64. Quoted in E.J. Hobsbawm, Labouring Men (1968), p. 117.
65. British Medical Journal, The Milk Supply of Large Towns (1904), p. 62.

9. FEEDING THE HUNGRY SCHOOLCHILD IN THE FIRST HALF OF THE TWENTIETH CENTURY

JOHN HURT

The 1906 Act

On 29 April 1908 L.A. Selby-Bigge, the permanent secretary to the Board of Education, drafted a memorandum on the Education (Provision of Meals) Act of 1906 for the guidance of his new political master Walter Runciman, who had replaced Augustine Birrell in the ministerial reshuffle following H.H. Asquith's acceptance of the premiership. 'The Board were intended by Parliament', Selby-Bigge wrote, 'to protect the ratepayer against the socialist proclivities of Local Education Authorities'. The parliamentary debates had stressed, he explained, that the Act was not one for supplementing outdoor relief but an educational one. Section 2 of the Act, requiring local authorities to recover the cost of meals provided for schoolchildren from their parents wherever possible, was more of a social measure designed to check pauperism than a financial one since 'the cost of recovery would probably swallow up all or nearly all the money recovered'(1). Views such as these affected the day-to-day working of the Act until well after the outbreak of the Second World War. Even then, despite the central government's concern to safeguard the health of the future generation by ensuring that they received a supplement to their normal rations, local officials and others still saw the provision of free or cheap meals and milk as an act of charity rather than as an instrument of national survival.

In common with many other social services, whether or not specifically intended for children, both the school meal service and the provision of milk in schools owed their origins to the initiative of private agencies. The first important

178

society, the Destitute Children's Dinner Society, was founded in 1864, six years before the establishment of the first school boards. When the new board schools began to have some of the poorest children of our cities sitting in their classrooms some teachers realized that they faced social problems as well as educational ones. Amongst the first to do so was Mrs. E.M. Burgwin, the newly appointed headmistress of Orange Street Board School, Southwark. Coming to the school from a more prosperous district she was so puzzled and disconcerted by the pallid appearance of the children that she sought medical advice only to be told that the children were severely undernourished. The efforts she and her staff made to give the children some extra food out of their own pockets eventually grew into the Referee Children's Free Dinner and Breakfast Fund thanks to the support she obtained from George Sims, a reporter on that newspaper(2). During the mid-1880s following the publication of Dr. Crichton-Browne's report on the alleged overpressure of work in public elementary schools, in which he drew attention to the inadequate diet of many of the children, and the severe winter of 1885-6 which intensified the current downward swing of the trade cycle, the number of voluntary organizations began to expand. Many of these bodies provided self-supporting meals, that is, they expected parents to pay at least the cost of the food provided. This attempt to ensure that the masses did not become pauperized soon proved nugatory; parents could not afford a farthing, let alone a penny, for the meals. They became free.

The voluntary societies relied on annual appeals in the newspapers around Christmas so that they could provide meals during the coldest months of the early New Year. Twenty years later another bad winter, that of 1904-5, reinforcing the downward swing of the economy following the cessation of the Boer War, led to renewed efforts to expand existing facilities. By the time the Education (Provision of Meals) Act received the Royal Assent charitable funds were providing around £30,000 a year. Contemporaneously the long and hard-fought campaign on the South African veldt had provided a traumatic experience for a people who prided themselves on possessing the largest empire the world had ever seen. The high rejection rate of volunteers for the colours gave substance to the view that the new cities of the nineteenth century

179

were the nurseries of a degenerate race(3). Yet
it required reports from the Royal Commission on
Physical Training (Scotland) in 1903, the question-
begging entitled Inter-Departmental Committee on
Physical Deterioration in 1904, the Inter-Departmental Committee on the Medical Inspection and
Feeding of Children Attending Public Elementary
Schools in 1905 and the Select Committee on Education (Provision of Meals) Bill of the following
year before a Liberal government set aside parliamentary time for the necessary legislation. The
new Act allowed local authorities to levy a halfpenny rate for the provision of school meals. Concern to ensure an effective way of distinguishing
between the 'deserving' and 'undeserving' poor,
anxiety lest the new legislation would open up
a Pandora's box of profligate public expenditure,
the bogey of socialism, and fears that the poor
would become dependent on the state for their
sustenance and progressively for all their material
needs were some of the issues that had made government action so hesitant.

Consequently the Board of Education was ever
at pains to emphasize that the Act was intended
neither to extend the existing provision of poor
relief nor to provide a substitute agency for its
distribution. The measure was an educational one
for 'any of those children attending a public
elementary school...unable by reason of lack of
food to take full advantage of the education
provided for them', a provision later repeated
in the consolidating Education Act of 1921. Although the Board relaxed its attitudes to some
extent in the late 1930s, it discouraged local
authorities from selecting children for free meals
by a means test throughout the inter-war years.
Such a procedure not only smacked of poor relief
but seemed to allow such children free meals as
of right. The selection of children was a matter
for the school medical officer. This made it an
educational measure in the eyes of the Board. Yet
the person best qualified to make the educational
judgement, the teacher, was not given a formal
place in the selection process until after the
inauguration of the milk in schools scheme.

Making a virtue out of this tortuous situation
the Board argued that medical selection brought
to light two categories of children that might
have remained undetected by the use of a means
test alone. First there were those children whose
parents' sense of shame would have stopped them

from revealing their poverty and applying for assistance under a means-test scheme. This argument could have been extended to having free meals at all as their very acceptance was a mark of poverty. The second group for whom the Board professed concern was those whose parents enjoyed higher incomes but who, through ignorance or indifference, failed to feed their offspring properly. However, the Board's real concern was to limit the number of applicants. Reliance on the medical officer, a memorandum of March 1928 pointed out, would enable local authorities to avoid having to feed all necessitous children or children of families that might qualify on an income basis. Moreover the Board could strengthen the hand of local authorities by making frequent visits to ensure that the Board's conditions and standards of nutrition were met. As Sir George Newman, chief medical officer of the Board of Education, minuted later the same year, medical selection was a method of sound administration. Its recent neglect had allowed school feeding to be so widely used as a relief measure.

The Board, fearing that the school meal service might be the thin edge of the socialist wedge, wanted to keep control in its own hands and those of the local authorities. Thus it opposed interference from outside politically or religiously-motivated welfare organizations, especially in such centres of political and religious dissent as South Wales. Somewhat paradoxically the same concern to limit the welfare role of the state led the Board to concede that those very authorities, whom it wanted to keep out of the soup kitchen, could be safely allowed to distribute boots and shoes. Local authority intervention in such a matter was fraught with danger for 'It would be a very serious departure for the Board or local authority to accept direct responsibility for securing that the children are properly clothed and shod, however logical an extension of compulsory education and the provision of meals this may be'(4).

The coal strikes of 1921 and 1926 together with the general strike in the latter year revived an issue first raised in 1912, that of the propriety of feeding strikers' children at public expense. Miners apparently regarded free school meals as one of the ways by which they could tide themselves over until they returned to work. In a number of instances they paid for the meals once a settlement was reached. The Nottingham miners ran up a bill for £2,025 in 1921 while those in Durham were still paying off their debts two or three years later(5). Unlike relief in kind from the poor law guardians school meals carried no taint of charity to men on strike prepared to pay later. Moreover after the 1921 strike ended local authorities did not cut back their services to their earlier levels. As a consequence 592,518 children received free meals at a cost of £983,182, albeit some of this money was later recovered, figures that showed more than a threefold increase on the previous year. Local authority estimates for 1922-3 of £636,472 were still more than double the exceptionally high year of 1920-1. After announcing a limit of £300,000 to the rate support grant the Board of Education introduced a rationing system based on the regional unemployment index figures, a measure that eventually brought the estimates down to £338,283. At this point it received Treasury approval to budget for £335,000 as 'the legality of our action in rationing this service has been challenged, and our legal position is shaky'(6).

The introduction of a rationing system implied that authorities would have to choose between one child 'unable by lack of food to take full advantage of the education provided' and another equally necessitous child. Not only was there no legal basis for such an action but there was no statutory justification for discriminating against children whose fathers were on strike. The cause of a child's destitution, whether it was chronic or temporary, did not come into the issue. From this it follows that the Board's attempts to distinguish between meals granted as an education measure and those given as a form of relief were equally without legal foundation.

Certainly the Board had had no such qualms in 1914. The lavish provision of school meals, far from demoralizing a society, was seen as a safeguard for its stability. On 4 August, the day war was declared, Sir George Newman drew the attention of J.A. Pease, President of the Board of Education, to the great social dislocation anticipated on the outbreak of war: 'Experience shows that food riots are inspired largely by the hunger of children; and if that problem can be met, a large operating factor in the causation of riots is removed '(7). On the same day the Education (Provision of Meals) Bill, removing the halfpenny limit to expenditure from the rates and allowing school meals to be provided in school holidays, passed the committee stage and received a hurried third reading in the House of Commons. The following day Earl Beauchamp, the Lord Privy Seal, indicated that the government wanted to speed it through the House of Lords: 'There may be grave danger of starvation in some of our large centres of population, and if this Bill becomes law it would be more easy to deal with school children'(8). The Bill received its second and third readings on 6 August and the Royal Assent the next day. That same day the Board issued a circular advising local authorities that they should establish machinery to deal with any emergency that might arise, so effectively had the invasion of Belgium temporarily stifled any fear of the onward march of socialism. Within a fortnight of the outbreak of war the Board had issued a circular introducing a rate support grant for school meals. The Board also envisaged the use of all 21,000 elementary-school premises for feeding children, the mobilization of school attendance officers and school nurses to assist the teachers, the abandonment of any form of selection, save that of necessity, and giving up any attempt to recover the cost of meals. In addition children below and above school age were to be eligible for meals. These groups were to be the financial responsibility of the local committee for the prevention and relief of distress, agencies under the control of a Central Advisory Committee chaired by Herbert Samuel, president of the Local Government Board. Although nearly 200,000 children received free meals at the beginning of October 1914, the numbers soon fell with the revival of the economy and the payment of marriage allowances to wives whose husbands had joined the armed forces(9).

The relief of distress in the 1920s

Despite the groundlessness of official fears of food riots in 1914, one member of the Board of Education recalled in 1922 how anxious they had been to pass the Bill as soon as possible to relieve the anticipated distress. By this time the political expediency of denying strikers' children school meals was under question. Only the previous year the Board had received reports that 'In more than one area disturbances were threatened unless meals were given to practically all the children whose parents were out of work.' On the basis of this experience an official predicted 'serious trouble if there is a strike in the mining areas and if no meals are forthcoming' when negotiations between men and masters were near breakdown in 1925. In July of the following year when the miners were on strike the President of the Board of Education warned the Cabinet that any attempt at rationing money to local authorities 'would do more harm than good'. Again official forebodings proved unjustified. So cautiously did the local authorities act in 1926, despite C.P. Trevelyan's removal of any limit on local authority expenditure in 1924, that they fed 200,000 fewer children at a cost of £150,000 less than in 1921, although the 1926 coal strike that lasted more than twice as long in some fields as the earlier one(10).

Another concern of inter-war governments was to prevent the granting of double relief, that is to stop children whose fathers received some form of unemployment relief that included maintenance for their children from having free meals as well. The Inter-Departmental Committee on Public Assistance, appointed by A. Bonar Law in 1923, made the 'special danger of overlapping between assistance under the School Meals Service in England and Wales and poor relief' one of its concerns. So many children had been fed in 1921 that 'the scheme was being improperly used as a means of relieving destitution', a judgement for which the relevant acts provided no justification. To prevent 'double relief' the Committee considered the 'adoption of a definite practice of giving a portion of...relief in the form of meals...highly desirable, in the interests both of the economical use of public funds and of the efficient feeding of the children'(11). The Report appeared in December 1923, the month of the downfall of Baldwin's government. Trevelyan, newly appointed as President of the Board of Education in J.R. MacDonald's first Labour government, concerned lest the Report's recommendation would limit the freedom of local authorities to feed children in a time of emergency, refused to implement it(12).

The two major strikes in the coalfields were symptoms of a greater malaise, the relative decline of the British coal industry in the inter-war years. Although outsiders might be struck by the unhealthy appearance of the children, doctors in daily contact with the long-term effects of poor diet grew accustomed to it. It required an outsider, such as the newly-appointed schools medical officer to Hebburn, county Durham, who in 1935 promptly found twice as many children as his predecessor in need of extra meals, to challenge locally-accepted standards(13). Such an action could raise an awkward problem. Low rateable values produced a low general-rate yield. In 1933-4 the products of a penny rate in terms of each elementary-school child in Merthyr Tydfil (general rate of 28s. 5d. in the £), Abertillery (29s. in the £) and Jarrow (19s. 6d. in the £) were 1s. 6d., 1s. 0d., and 1s. 2d. respectively. In the more prosperous seaside resorts of Bournemouth (7s. 4d. in the £), Hove (7s. 6d. in the £) and Blackpool (7s. 6d. in the £) with a comparatively elderly population the yields were 14s. 5d., 19s. 6d., and 11s. 4½d. respectively. Thus in Pontypridd (23. 11d. in the £), for example, the provision of free milk, biscuits, and cod liver oil alone put 3½d. on the rates. Poor authorities faced a further difficulty. As a family's first charge on its budget was that of meeting its rent and rates the cost of any extension of the school meals service would have brought those families just above the poverty line into the poverty trap. Unable to claim free meals for their own children, they would have had to feed them from an insufficient housekeeping allowance further reduced by higher rates. In addition, the tradition whereby the adequate feeding of the breadwinning father was the first dietary consideration of mining families still persisted to the detriment of the interests of the children(14). Local authorities had the further problem of deciding where their priorities lay at a time when they were committed to the expense of the reorganization of secondary education. In 1926, for example, Lord Eustace Percy, President of the Board of Education, had equated the cost of feeding the miners' children that year with that of rebuilding schools for 25,000 children 'now taught in schools which were scarcely fit to house a pig'. Alternatively the money could have provided secondary-school accommodation for 8,000 more children(15).

There can be little doubt that the Board of Education played down the gravity of the situation in the worst years of the depression in the distressed areas. By advocating the selection of children on medical criteria and discouraging the use of a means test the proportion of children receiving free meals of any description, breakfasts, dinners, milk, teas, cod liver oil, dried milk

185

and various proprietary foods seldom exceeded 8
per cent of the average attendance in England and
Wales. Although the ensuing tension was greatest
in areas of poverty and high unemployment where
the Labour party was well represented at both local
and national levels, these were the very areas
that lacked the resources to implement the social
services their local leaders would have liked to
have had. Hence the Board at times had to urge
local authorities even in Labour strongholds to
make greater effort. At the same time it had to
rebut criticisms from the political right of con-
doning extravagance.

The Board also took care to avoid publicity
where possible. Following the receipt of a report
made by two of the Board's doctors that 'things
were...on the verge of collapse' in South Wales,
Lord Eustace Percy visited the area for himself.
The Board managed to keep the news of his visit
out of the press(16). Similarly, the Board vetoed
a proposed visit by local medical officers to London
as 'it would only cause a great deal too much talk
in South Wales where the Trade and Labour Councils
were already beginning to agitate for school feeding'. The one positive step to assist the children
of South Wales came the following winter when a
grant from the Lord Mayor of London's Coalfields
Distress Appeal Fund enabled the local authorities
there and in the North-East to increase the number
of children fed from 9,475 to 22,148(17). Slight
though this help may have been, it came at a time
when the leading newspapers, including The Times
had refused to publish a letter from the Save the
Children Fund to assist the children of the depressed areas(18).

The school milk scheme

Although the attitudes described above survived
the outbreak of the Second World War, the inauguration of the Milk in Schools Scheme in 1934, 'the
largest experiment in supplementary school feeding
the world has yet seen', marked the beginning of
an expansionist and more liberal phase. The primum
mobile of the scheme was Walter Elliot's concern
to assist dairy farmers facing the problem of overproduction. Recognizing that 'The purpose of
Elliot's scheme seems to be to divert surplus milk
from the butter and cheese factories to the liquid
milk market', the Board of Education quickly vetoed
Elliot's suggestion that 5 million children should

have a third of a pint a day and thereby consume 45 million gallons a year. If every child were to have milk every day it would have to be free. This the Board could not accept: 'It is a well established and accepted principle that those parents who can afford it should pay for medical treatment and feeding of their children. A general supply of free milk might well lead to demands for the free supply of medical treatment and school dinners.' Similarly secondary-school pupils were ruled out of court because of the 'different conditions and the generally better financial status of the parents'. To avoid any laxity over the provision of school meals the Board contemplated asking for an amendment to the 1921 Act to allow local authorities to provide milk, but not other meals, for any poor child, without regard to any question of malnutrition, a move the Treasury vetoed(19).

The expectation that the excess supply of milk over demand would reach 40 per cent by the summer of 1934 thereby endangering the price structure of the market had led to Elliot's initiative at the end of 1933. Only shortly before, in the winter of 1932-3, the agricultural price index had reached its inter-war nadir when it stood only a few points above the pre-war level. Yet this had occurred at a time of low production following the unfortunate summers of 1929 and 1931, one a drought and the other possibly the wettest and coldest since that of 1879(20).

From 1922 onwards the Permanent Joint Milk Committee had operated a differential price system under which farmers received one price for milk sold for manufacturing purposes, i.e. making butter, cheese, cream, condensed milk, plastics, and etc., and a higher price for milk sold for human consumption. By 1933, the year in which the Milk Marketing Board was formed, the price the farmer received for manufacturing milk had fallen from 8½d. a gallon in 1928 to 5d. and even 4¾d. Yet the price of milk sold to the public had remained remarkably stable. A high-cost form of distribution, which in London included two deliveries a day, overlapping rounds and the use of half-pint bottles, justified in the retailers' minds their margin of 9d. to 1s. a gallon, an amount that doubled the price of milk between the farmer and the doorstep(21).

Unfortunately for the farmer and the health of the nation fresh milk did not reach every doorstep every day. A Ministry of Agriculture Report published in 1935 suggested that the average per capita consumption of milk was between 1/3 and 2/5ths of a pint a day, a figure that concealed variations ranging from 0.68 pints in Bournemouth to 0.22 pints in Hull. A survey of households in Cardiff found a positive correlation between the consumption of fresh milk and social class and an inverse one for skimmed milk. The average consumption of fresh milk in good middle-class households was 3.8 pints and of skimmed milk 0.25 pints; in working-class homes containing children but which were not slums, the corresponding figures were 1.1 and 3.24 pints. Yet children in only four of the thirty-one homes surveyed had any milk at school(22). Poorer homes supplemented their fresh milk with sweetened condensed milk, a product that had two advantages over the former. It kept better in hot weather in homes that in the 1930s would not have possessed refrigerators. If diluted to the same consistency as fresh milk it was a cheaper substitute. Moreover if money ran out towards the end of week further economies could be made by still further dilution. With such a flexibly priced alternative to fresh milk and given the price inelasticity of the latter, which had nòt fallen in line with other agricultural products, the farmer's prospects of selling his summer surplus for human consumption were bleak(23).

The Milk Act of 1934 subsidized the price of milk over the next two years at a cost of £3,000,000 to £3,500,000, provided £750,000 for improving dairy herds and gave £1,000,000 for encouraging the consumption of fresh milk partly by publicity measures and partly by the Milk in Schools Scheme. The Act was renewed and extended in scope by further ones in 1937, 1938, and 1939. Modest as the original Act was, it only obtained Treasury sanction after some misgiving. Neville Chamberlain, then Chancellor of the Exchequer, only agreed when he was convinced that there was no other way of securing a large increase in the consumption of milk. He also found 'a most awkward possibility...any suggestion that the government are pursuing a policy of supplying, or subsidizing the supply of, extra quantities of free milk, because the precedent can so easily be extended to other food, clothes etc.' The Treasury accordingly had opposed any change to the Education Act of 1921 that would have allowed children to be selected on an income basis. Such a procedure would be 'most dangerous' as it might be interpreted as subsidizing the price of milk to the consumer(24). Although the bill reflected the enlightened paternalism of the Conservative landed interest, it drew criticism from some of the party's back-benchers for subsidizing both the production and the consumption of milk. However the distribution of cheap and free milk through the schools prevented it from reaching the general public.

The development of the Milk in Schools Scheme had followed a pattern common to many other social services; the government was giving official support to one already in existence. Although children had been given milk before the 1906 Act, such efforts had been purely local in character. The formation of the National Milk Publicity Council in 1920 marks the start at a national level of an organized attempt to boost the sale of milk to adults and children alike. In the autumn of that year Dr. G.A. Auden, medical officer of health for Birmingham, carried out a small-scale experiment in assessing the nutritional benefit of giving poor children milk daily, the results of which were published under the title, A Notable Experiment in the Feeding of Children (1922). By 1929 some 500,000 children were paying the normal retail price of a penny for a third of a pint. In addition local authorities provided up to 500,000 free milk meals a week. Even a pint of milk for threepence cost local authorities less than a solid meal which had to bear extra costs of cooking and administration. In nutritional terms it compared favourably with a solid meal. A pint of milk offered 378 kilocalories and 18.7 grams of first-class protein whereas it is unlikely that all school dinners met the London County Council's target of 750 kcals and 25g. of first-class protein(25).

Although the child sucking his milk through his straw had become a familiar sight in the classroom by 1934, the new scheme halving the cost of milk to the paying consumer was launched amid a fanfare of publicity. Walter Elliot, the minister responsible, made a broadcast in which he thought it necessary to lay the ghost of the workhouse and begrudging charity of the past by reassuring parents that just because the milk was cheap it was not inferior. It was 'exactly the same good milk that is available now, with the added security of the school Medical Officer's certificate, and the County Medical Officer over that'. On 1 October, the first day of the new scheme, Elliot made a ministerial visit to an elementary school of the L.C.C. to see children having their milk. Elliot's target of three million children drinking milk by the following Easter was not realized until the third year of the Second World War(26). As fresh cows' milk did not form an important part of working-class diet many children found the experience of drinking cold milk strange and distasteful as it lacked the sweetening of the more familiar condensed variety. Children, and parents who found pasteurized milk a novelty, complained that it tasted burnt and was less wholesome than raw milk. Farmers, who had previously sold their milk raw, complained that they were debarred from contracts under the new scheme(27). In some rural areas small schools did not join the scheme as local roundsmen found their retailer's margin too small to justify the necessary capital outlay in cleaning machinery and the special sized bottles. By March 1939 there were still 13.1 per cent of all elementary school departments, containing 5 per cent of the school population, mainly in rural areas, outside the scheme. Of the children in schools within the scheme, but not having free milk, 53.4 per cent were paying their daily half-penny(28).

In introducing the scheme the Board of Education made the seemingly generous gesture that it would 'regard as proper that children should be selected who show any symptoms, however slight, of subnormal nutrition'. The further stipulation that 'the selection of children for free meals should be by a system of medical inspection by the Authority's Medical Officers' virtually nullified this apparent magnaminity. As the national health service did not cover a worker's dependants there could be long gaps in a child's life when he never saw a doctor of any description apart from the school doctor who gave him a cursory examination three times in his school career. Fifteen months later, in December 1935, the Board gave a qualified approval to the use of means tests. 'The Board saw no reason generally to question the reasonableness of the income scales adopted by Authorities normally fixed high enough to cover those whose parents were receiving unemployment allowances or working for low wages'(29). The Board also sanctioned the gratuitous feeding of children while they were waiting to be seen by a doctor. In addition local authorities were encouraged to open wider their nets by inviting reports from teachers, nurses, attendance officers,

and others on children who might benefit from free
milk. To cope with the medical examination of
these extra children the Board suggested more
frequent medical inspections than the three statutory ones. The introduction of the Milk in Schools Scheme
put a burden on existing selection procedures at
a time when not only was their efficacy being
challenged but the state of the nation's health
was becoming a matter for informed public debate.
The Board's guarded approval of the use of income
scales came just one year after the appearance
of the British Medical Association's Report on
Nutrition which revealed the gap between the
'minimum weekly expenditure required on foodstuffs...if health and working capacity are to
be maintained' and the income available to the
unemployed and lowly-paid worker. Taking the
B.M.A.'s figures for food and those of the Social
Survey of Merseyside for fuel, clothing, lighting,
and heating, a man and his wife on maximum benefit
had a surplus of 9s. 4d. a week with which to meet
all other expenses. A married couple with three
children under the age of ten had a surplus of
2s.3d. while a family with five children, admittedly
a demographic rarity, started with a deficit of
5s. 3d. before they met any other expenses. Although
the U.A.B. benefit was only 2s. a child a week,
the B.M.A. had been unable to prepare a diet for
a child that cost less than half-a-crown. Moreover,
the food necessary and suitable for a young child
was relatively more expensive per unit of energy
than that for older children and adults. The
Report was criticized in the B.M.A's Journal for
citing unrealistically low prices and for the
insufficiency of the diet used. For instance,
between the making of the survey and its publication, the Milk Marketing Board had fixed the
minimum price of milk at 3½d., a three-farthings
rise on the figure the B.M.A. used. By late 1937
the position had deteriorated still further. Whereas
the cost of the B.M.A's diet had been 22s. 6½d.
in 1933, a survey of November 1937 suggested that
a more realistic figure was 29s. 6d. to 30s. 6d.,
a calculation that still only allowed 2s. 6d.,
the 1933 amount, for fresh fruit and vegetables(30).
        Other surveys including J.B. Orr, Food, Health
and Income (1936), Colin Clark, The National Income
(1937) and a series of locally-based ones underlined
the conclusions one could draw from the B.M.A.
Report on Nutrition. Although Sir (later Lord)

John Boyd Orr's verdict that 10 per cent of the
population, including 20 to 25 per cent of the
country's children, had a diet deficient in every
constituent examined, and that less than 50 per
cent could be safely regarded as adequately fed
'for the maintenance of perfect health' was
challenged on the grounds of the rigorous criteria
used, later criticisms did little to blunt the
earlier impact of his findings. Colin Clark in
The National Income, for example, put 25.3 per
cent of the nation's children in families with
a per capita income of less than 10s., the amount
required for full health. In local studies, the
proportion of children in working-class families
below an income line drawn more stringently than
that of the B.M.A. was 24.5 per cent in Liverpool,
30 per cent in Southampton, 26.9 per cent
in Sheffield, and 39 per cent in Miles Platting,
Manchester. A further survey made by Women's Section of the Labour Party in 1936 found 15 per cent
of all children in 1,000 poor working-class homes
seriously underfed and another 20 per cent insuf-
ficiently fed(31). Two other publications reflect
the extent of public concern about the state of
the nation's health and the contemporary fear that
Great Britain might become a C3 nation unable to
defend herself. These were the First Report of
the Ministry of Health's Advisory Committee on
Nutrition (1937), probably 'the first comprehensive
survey, statistical and physiological, of the diet
of a whole nation set on foot by any government'(32)
and Britain's Health (Penguin Books, 1939) a summary
for a wider readership of the P.E.P. Report on
the British Health Services.
     After the outbreak of war, B. Seebohm Rowntree
published his Poverty and Progress (1941) based
on a survey of York made in 1936 after the worst
of the depression was over. Rowntree found 31.1
per cent of the working-class population, 17.8
per cent of the total population of the city, living
below a poverty line based on the B.M.A.'s minimum
recommended diet. Of the 17,185 persons below
this level, 5,776 were children under the age of
14 who formed 28.2 per cent of the city's children.
Yet the notional value of the free milk and meals
the children in this group received represented
no more than £15 12s. 9d. of the total income of
£8,928 9s. 11d. of this section of York's
citizens(33).
     If one accepts the cumulative evidence of
the various surveys made in the 1930s as reliable

there can be no doubting the inadequacy of the
provision made for providing poor children with
free meals and milk. In 1938, when the number
of insured workers registered as unemployed stood
at 1,810,000, there were still 47 of the 315 local
education authorities making no attempt to provide
any form of free meals. Expressed as percentages
of the total average attendance of children in
England and Wales, 11.5 per cent received free
milk only; 1.2 per cent free meals only; and 2.8
per cent both free meals and free milk. During
the decade local authorities had been readier to
expand the milk service, because of its relative
cheapness and administrative convenience, than
the meal service. In 1938 some 635,174 children
received free milk as compared with 36,000 in 1930.
In 1932 there were 900,000 paying the full price
for milk and over 2,500,000 having it at half price
in 1938. By contrast, the number of free solid
meals had increased only slowly from 26,471,520
to 26,819,108 served to 176,767 children in 1938.
In one respect the official statistics present
an unduly rosy picture for they refer to individual
children: the daily average number of children
taking free milk and meals in 1938 was nearer
560,000 and 110,000. In other words the provision
of free meals was not seen as a regular practice
but only as a temporary expedient for the particular
child(34).

The contrast between the findings of independent social investigators and the practice of local
authorities brought criticism both from the political left, stirred by a concern for the welfare
of the underprivileged, and the political right,
prompted by anxieties about national defence, who
found common ground in wanting to improve the welfare services available to the young. Moreover
the pressures that had prompted the Milk in Schools
Scheme and the Drink More Milk Campaign were
expansionist whereas the assumption underlying
the Board of Education's commitment to the assessment of children by medical examination was restrictive. The fall in the birth rate to 15.8 by 1931
not only provided the basis for a number of gloomy
projections about the future size of the population
but also justified a policy of enhancing
the physical well-being of the nation's youth,
an issue on which there was a measure of agreement
across the political parties(35).

A Conservative speaker summed up this attitude
early in 1936: 'If the standard of nutrition of

the whole population were brought up to that even
now attained in a lower middle-class household,
there would be...an immense reinforcement of the
nation's power to survive periods of stress.'
The Spanish civil war began the following summer.
Against this background, Neville Chamberlain's
speech to the Conservative Party Conference in
September, in which he referred to the need to
take steps to improve the national physique, was
well received. He wrote in his diary afterwards:
'The main result of taking this meeting appears
to be a general acceptance of my position as heir
apparent [to Stanley Baldwin] and acting P.M.'(36)
Favourable reactions from the press encouraged
the government under his leadership to proceed
with the Physical Training and Recreation Act the
following session. The government, disavowing
any intention of copying Germany or Italy or of
having militarist intentions claimed that recent
improvements in the school curriculum for physical
education had created a demand for better sports
facilities for those who had recently left
school(37). Yet the new syllabus was only three
years old and the provision of such additional
resources as an increased supply of teachers trained
in physical education and more gymnasia and playing
fields still in its infancy. The appearance in
the following year of Recreation and Physical Fitness for Girls and Young Women and the complementary
Recreation and Physical Fitness for Youths and
Young Men was a tacit acceptance of the Board of
Education's responsibilities to those who had left
school. Before this time there was little supplementary provision for infants and young people
outside the normal range of school years. The
Maternity and Child Welfare Act, 1918, under which
local authorities could provide cheap or free milk
to nursing mothers and infants was virtually a
dead letter. Those who had just left school benefited from the extension of the national health
insurance to include the fourteen to sixteen year
olds in 1938. If they were unemployed and attending
a Juvenile Instruction Centre they were eligible
under certain conditions to have free milk from
1934 onwards, a scheme that the Unemployment Insurance Act put on a more liberal basis in 1938.
        Against a background of factors making for
a more liberal welfare policy the selection of
children on medical grounds lost such clinical
credibility as it once possessed. Even the files
of the Board of Education on the depressed areas,

although generally supportive of the thesis that
no more than 5 per cent of the children needed
extra nourishment, at times reveal an underlying
disquiet. In a general report on South Wales,
Dr. J.E. Underwood, one of the Board of Education's
doctors, accepted the standard figure for under-
nourishment as around 4 to 5 per cent but also
wrote of 'the general lassitude of children in
the coalmining areas which official statistics
of malnutrition hid'. In his opinion: 'with the
present arrangements for feeding school children
we are only just staving off a deterioration in
health and physique, and therefore the necessity
of keeping these arrangements working at full
pressure' remained. When shown a report assessing
240 of 749 infants as undernourished, he admitted
that his own examinations had been cursory and
that the children were neither stripped nor weighed.
If he had examined the children more carefully
his own conclusions 'would have almost certainly
approximated more closely to those of Dr. Jones'
whose survey he had been shown(38).
    The B.M.A.'s Report on Nutrition of 1933 raised
the issue publicly:

> The Committee...desires to place on record
> its regret that there exists no satisfactory
> and accepted routine method by which the
> nutritional condition or state of individuals
> can be assessed, and by which the findings
> of different observers can be compared. The
> absence of a satisfactory standard of 'normal
> nutrition' is probably the explanation why
> so many divergent opinions are expressed as
> to the nutritional condition of...school chil-
> dren. The usually adopted age, height, and
> weight ratios are open to serious objection
> when applied to individuals.

Apart from having to examine many more children
than before, the start of the Milk in Schools Scheme
added to the doctors' clinical dilemma in other
ways. Although children were eligible for free
milk if they showed 'any symptoms, however slight,
of subnormal nutrition' signs of incipient malnutrition were very difficult to detect. In addition it was bad preventive practice to wait for
clinical evidence which would bear scientific
scrutiny before authorizing free milk. As one
school medical officer successfully argued, such
a course of action lacked legal justification:

195

'There is nothing in the 1921 Act about a trial period of starvation... The proper selection is of children who suffer from lack of food...the only condition laid down in the Act... Why, then, does the Board insist...that the child must wait till the lack of food actually produces diagnosable malnutrition'(39).

Despite these criticisms from the medical profession the Board held to its belief that malnutrition could be detected by a simple medical examination until the publication of R.H. Jones's article, 'Physical Indices and Clinical Assessment of the Nutrition of Schoolchildren' in the Journal of the Royal Statistical Society in early 1938. Jones analysed the findings of a number of controlled experiments to show the subjective nature of doctors' assessments of children and the extent to which apparent agreement by medical practitioners about the percentage of a particular group of children requiring additional feeding masked differences of opinion over the condition of individual ones(40). The Board of Education perforce admitted that there was 'no accepted objective method of measuring malnutrition' and that 'clinical assessment was very fallible'(41).

In the same year it reported: 'The provision of free meals is unduly restricted by the operation of a severe income scale, which has often been in force for many years without alteration.' The Board wrote to about 150 local authorities suggesting improvements in provision, more lenient scales, and improved methods of selection. Whereas at the start of the inter-war years their concern had been to restrict the feeding services by 1939 the Board's officials were chivying the wayward. For example, unable to accept the finding that only 2.4 per cent of Mountain Ash's children required additional feeding, they sent two of their own officials who put 19.6 per cent of the children in the poorer schools in that category and another 16 per cent on the borderline. A further survey made in Swansea, where the Board had protested at the stringency of the income scales, found 7,580 children requiring extra food but only 280 having free dinners and 3,500 free milk(42).

The appointment of a dietician to the Board of Education in the spring of 1938 was yet another belated reform but portent of future good intent. Of the 66 authorities she visited in her first year of office she found only 5 per cent were making really good arrangements while 20 per cent were

entirely unsatisfactory(43). At one West Riding
centre where there were no green vegetables on
the menu, the children 'ate their food like little
wild animals' with their filthy hands. At another
the same bones were boiled three days a week to
provide soup. A third centre changed the newspapers on the tables every other day and served
a thin soup made in a wash boiler before being
poured into a slop pail and then ladled into the
children's plates(44).
A few months before the outbreak of war the
Board prepared an estimate of the cost of putting
eligibility for school meals on an income basis.
Using the B.M.A.'s report of 1933, with adjustments
for subsequent price rises some 1,300,000 children,
at a time when less than a tenth of that number
received free meals daily, were thought to be
eligible. Allowing 6d. a head, 3½d. for food and
2½d. for overheads - a recognition of the inadequacy
of the current 2.94d. on food for each meal - the
estimated cost was £6,500,000 for 200 schooldays
a year and £9,750,000 if holidays were included(45).
Thus although much remained to be done to extend
the scope of the social services in the schools
by the time war came The Times could write, with
greater justification than would have been possible
twenty years earlier: 'Schools have to do more
than merely train the mind and the body of the
child; they have to eradicate the results of last
century's hectic industrialization. They are not
only educating; they are also performing a great
eugenic function and rectifying some of the great
social injustices of the past'(46).

Expansion during the Second World War

The evacuation of three-quarters of a million
children from British cities at the outbreak of
war was a success in logistics. Nutritionally,
it was a disaster for those poor children who moved
from authorities that provided welfare food services
to those that did not. Those children who stayed
behind may have rejoiced at the closing of their
schools but hunger soon blunted their sense of
euphoria. Local authorities in the reception areas
justified their failure to organize free meal services on the grounds that the billeting allowance
covered the full cost of board. Landladies argued
that the billeting allowance was insufficient for
them to pay out for meals or milk at school. By
October 1939 the number of children receiving free

meals had fallen to its lowest level for fifty years. Although there was then some revival, the numbers of children taking free meals and milk in July 1940, 130,000 and 2,100,000 respectively, were still below those for the last months of peace(47).

By this time, the first of four wartime moves to expand the school meal service was under way. The German occupation of the Low Countries, the evacuation of the British army from the Continent, and the French armistice signed on 22 June raised the possibility of a widespread bomber offensive against this country followed by an invasion and its attendant disruption of the public utilities serving the civilian population. Meanwhile Clement Attlee, Lord Privy Seal, had already taken the initiative by looking at the problem of 'The Provision of Cheap Food for the Poorer Classes' or 'how to get the right food in the right quantities in the right stomachs'. As part of this plan he wanted school meals available to all irrespective of income. A few days later he suggested to H. Ramsbotham, President of the Board of Education, that the present provision of meals for 300,000 children out of 5,000,000 be considerably extended. The Ministry of Food also drafted a policy document for the Food and Policy Committee of the War Cabinet dealing with meals for war workers in factories and 'children...and nursing mothers whom, on grounds both of humanity and racial preservation, it is essential to protect against malnutrition, and those on lower incomes.' For this purpose the provision of milk was not enough. It was further pointed out that schools could be used as communal feeding centres for the population as a whole in the event of emergency. The use of other facilities such as hotels, restaurants, and large stores including Marks and Spencers and Woolworths was also advocated. In this way the question of extending the school meal service became part of a greater issue, that of providing communal feeding centres. On 24 June the Food and Policy Committee endorsed these proposals pointing out the ensuing savings of food and labour by developing communal feeding facilities. It further advocated the early implementation of the scheme to forestall any future disruption by accustoming people to the idea of communal feeding. As the 'social habits of the people would have to be modified', manipulation of the rationing system could serve as a means of indirect coercion(48).

With the somewhat reluctant agreement of the
Treasury the grant to local authorities was raised
from a scale varying between 6 per cent and 71
per cent to a minimum of 50 per cent and a maximum
of 92 per cent. Despite this financial encouragement, local authorities were slow to act. They
found British restaurants, which attracted a 100
per cent grant and charged prices to cover their
running costs, a much more attractive proposition.
By the autumn of 1941 there were still only about
300,000 children receiving school dinners either
free or for payment. With the meat ration cut
to 1d. a meal it was 'scarcely possible for school
canteens to offer dinners of a quality which could
be defended as satisfactory for the main meal of
the day for children'(49).
Meanwhile the development of the Milk
in Schools Scheme had made much more satisfactory
progress. The Ministry of Health's plan to give
mothers and infants cheap or free milk under the
Milk Industry Act, 1939, at first seemed as moribund
as that of the Maternity and Child Welfare Act,
1918. In July 1940 the latter scheme together
with another under which the Milk Marketing Board
had made cheap milk available in the depressed
areas were combined into the National Milk Scheme,
control of which now came under the Ministry of
Food. Within two months 70 per cent of the mothers
and infants eligible were having free or subsidized
milk. Middle-class mothers had taken advantage
of the offer thereby ridding it of the taint of
charity or poor relief that still stigmatized free
school dinners. Whereas the pre-war problem had
been one of overproduction the wartime one was
one of supply. Mothers, schoolchildren, and infants
became priority consumers. By February the number
of children taking milk in schools was 2,479,000,
close to the pre-war figure. By the autumn the
number had increased to over 3,000,000, the target
Walter Elliot had set in 1934, and more than 75
per cent of the school population. The figure
remained around 3,300,000 for the rest of the war,
a stability that conceals an increase in the
proportion of children having two-thirds of a pint
from 19 per cent in February 1941 to 40 per cent
shortly before D-Day, June 1944(50).
Higher infantile mortality and tuberculosis
rates, together with the realization that children
from comfortable as well as poor families were
suffering from an inadequate diet provided the
background to a Cabinet decision to expand the

school meal service in the autumn of 1941. As a corollary to the growing assumption that the war was being fought for the benefit of the common people the government assumed a greater responsibility for their welfare. 'I want', said Lord Woolton, Minister for Food, 'to see elementary school children as well fed as children going to Eton and Harrow. I am determined that we shall organize our food front that at the end of the war, unlike the last, we shall have preserved and even improved the health and physique of the nation'(51). Children were at last able to have cheap meals without being both necessitous and undernourished. The government announced extra financial support for local authorities, the use of emergency cooking centres set up after the air raids on provincial cities earlier the same year, and an improved scale of rations. School canteens, now run on a par with those providing for heavy workers in specified industries, had the meat ration doubled to 2d. a meal. Meals were to give 1,000 kcals to older children, an improvement on the L.C.C.'s target of 750 kcals set in 1916 which had become the norm for most authorities before 1939. The level of 1,000 kcals, which held the field from 1941 onwards, received general endorsement in 1975 when a sliding scale of 530 to 1,000 kcals for children aged 3 to 18 years was recommended(52).

Children received their meals from kitchens on school premises doubling up as emergency feeding centres, from British Restaurants, or from emergency feeding centres built to cope with civilian disruption following air raids. The 300 emergency centres, never fully used for their original purpose, supplied a peak of 200,000 meals a day in September 1943, a fifth of all school meals. From October onwards local authorities began to take over control of them from the Ministry of Food until the latter held no more than 50 in 1947(53).

The drive initiated in the autumn of 1941 reached its target of a million dinners a day within a year. In May 1943, the month of the heaviest shipping losses in either of the wars against Germany, war socialism took a further step forward. The Treasury announced a 100 per cent equipment grant thereby putting school canteens at last on a par with British Restaurants and emergency feeding centres. To assist their speedy building the Ministry of Works made priority allocations of equipment. Although preparations for the Second

Front and need to repair buildings after the flying bomb and rocket bomb offensive delayed the necessary construction work, by October 1945 39.7 per cent of school children were taking school dinners, a figure well short of the 75 per cent target of May 1943(54). The Education Act of the following year plugged the main gaps in earlier legislation. The provision of school meals and milk, previously a power that not every local education authority exercised, became a duty. Authorities now had to employ a school meals organizer. Despite wartime efforts to improve standards it was still possible to find authorities serving a meal of a quality and under conditions that were more of a deterrent than an incentive to either child or parent. An official visit to Bradford, a city with a long and honourable record in the provision of school meals, found the energy value of the meals to be 711 instead of 1,000 kcals with comparable deficiencies in protein and fat. At one canteen children ate corned beef with their fingers for there were no knives. The meal supervised by non-teaching staff was disorderly: 'The women helpers do their best to maintain order but their methods of shouting and banging on the table are not very efficient and cannot claim to be cultural'(55). Subsequent regulations prevented local authorities from charging more than the actual cost of the food, a power they had previously possessed but not always exercised. From August 1946 milk became free for all pupils attending grant-aided schools and independent ones, the latter having been admitted into the milk scheme in August 1942. Such was the sense of national unity in the immediate post-war era that the Report of the Committee on Milk Distribution (1948) looked to the day when every child would have two-thirds of a pint a day, the amount recommended by a League of Nations technical committee in the early 1930s, an objective still unachieved when the first cuts came in 1971(56).

NOTES

1. Public Record office, Ed. 50/8, 'Selby-Bigge to the President of the Board of Education, 29 April 1908'. In the period 1913-23 £159,838 was recovered from parents. This includes payments made by parents of non-necessitous children.
2. The early history of the school meal service

is more fully described in J.S. Hurt, Elementary Schooling and the Working Classes, 1860-
1918 (1979), Chapter V and pp. 145-52.

3. For a survey of the literature on this theme
see D.A. Reeder, 'Predicaments of City Children: late Victorian and Edwardian Perspectives
on Education and Urban Society', in D.A.
Reeder, Urban Education in the Nineteenth
Century (1977), pp. 75-94.

4. P.R.O, Ed. 50/83, 'Memorandum of 20 March
1928'; 'Sir George Newman's minute of 4 June
1928'.

5. The Times, 29 August, 1921; P.R.O., T172/1535,
'Pres. of the Board to the Cabinet, 15 July
1926'. I am indebted to Dr. W.R. Garside
for this reference.

6. The Health of the School Child, Annual Report
of the Chief Medical Officer of the Board
of Education for the Year 1922 (1923), pp.
117-8; P.R.O. Ed. 50/1372, 'Historical Note,
1906-1923, Memorandum prepared by M. Branch,
26 January 1923'. P.R.O, Ed. 24/1373, 'Selby-
Bigge to Sir George Barstow, Treasury, 14
December 1922'.

7. P.R.O, Ed. 24/1371, 'Sir George Newman to
A.J. Pearse, 4 August 1914'.

8. Hansard Fifth Series, Vol. XVII, c. 387, House
of Lords Debates, 5 August 1914.

9. Board of Education Circulars, 854 of 7 August
1914 and 856 of 15 August 1914. The latter
contains a number of specimen menus for large-
scale catering.

10. P.R.O, Ed. 50/1372, 'A.H. Wood's memorandum
on the provision of meals by L.E.A's in times
of special industrial disturbance, 20 July
1925'; P.R.O, T172/1535 op.cit.; Health of
the School Child, 1927 (1928), pp. 101-2.

11. Inter-Departmental Committee on Public Assistance Administration (Cmd. 2011, 1924), pp.
54-5.

12. Hansard Fifth Series, Vol. CLXIX, c. 1010,
House of Commons Debates, 14 February 1924.

13. M.E. Green, Malnutrition amongst School Children (1938), p. 7.

14. Children's Minimum Council, Special Areas
Bill, Memorandum on Proposed Provision for
Additional Food etc. for Mothers and Children
in Distressed Areas (1937), pp. 11-12.

15. The Times, 9 November, 1926.

16. The Times did not report the visit. It is
clear from Lord Percy's House of Commons

speech, Hansard Fifth Series, Vol. CCXV, c. 937-42, 26 March 1926, that the visit had recently taken place.

17. Health of the School Child, 1928 (1929), p.71.

18. P.R.O, Ed. 50/83, 'R.S. Wood's memorandum of 13 January 1928'.

19. P.R.O, Ed. 24/1367, 'Milk in School Proposal, H. Ramsbotham, 13 December 1933'; 'Note of discussion between President of the Board of Ed. and Minister of Agriculture, 15 December 1933'; 'Provision of Milk in School, unsigned, 20 February 1934'; 'C.L. Stocks (Treasury) to E.G. Howarth (Board of Ed.), letter of 1 March 1934'.

20. E.H. Whetham, The Agricultural History of England and Wales Vol. VIII, 1914-39 (1978),pp. 229-31. The growth of road transport widened the market for the milk producer. The prospect of a monthly milk cheque attracted him into it. Larger herds, improved lactation, and the decline of home farm butter and cheese making, in face of foreign imports, contributed to the problem of overproduction.

21. E.H. Whetham, op.cit., pp. 251-2; Ministry of Agriculture and Fisheries, Report of the Reorganization Commission for Milk, Economic Series No. 38 (1933), pp. 34-9, 60-2.

22. Reorganization Commission for Milk, p. 36. Hansard Fifth Series, Vol. CCXC, c. 388-90, House of Commons Debate, 31 May 1934.

23. With a recent rise in imports of cheese and butter from the British Empire the farmer's prospects in the manufacturing market were equally bleak as the Ottawa agreement of 1932 precluded the imposition of any restriction on this rapidly developing trade.

24. P.R.O, Ed. 50/81, 'Note of discussion between Walter Elliot and Milk Marketing Board, 22 February 1934'; 'Treasury to Board of Ed. 1 March 1934'. In December 1934 the cost of providing free milk on a means test basis was estimated to be £200,000 a year. Of the 25 per cent of elementary children who would have been eligible 10 per cent were already receiving it on medical grounds leaving 15 per cent not taking milk because their parents could not afford to pay a halfpenny a day. P.R.O, Ed. 50/82, 'Minute of 17 December 1934'. The same file contains a letter from King George V dated 15 January 1935, supporting the provision of free milk for poor children.

25. In one experiment children had fared better on half a pint a day than on either school dinners or home feeding, Health of the School Child, 1924 (1925), pp. 132-3: 'One important factor in maintaining the health of the school children is, undoubtedly the action of the Education Authorities in considerably extending the issue of free milk to children. At the end of 1933, 688 children were receiving free milk and biscuits with a special fat content. These are given instead of providing school meals.' Ministry of Labour Reports of Investigations into the Industrial Conditions in Certain Depressed Areas, I, West Cumberland and Haltwistle (1934). I am indebted to Mrs. G.M. Hurt for this reference.

26. Listener, 3 October 1934; The Times, 2 October 1934.

27. Lord Rowallan, President of the British Dairy Farmers' Association, complained 'they felt very strongly that they were being attacked by the medical profession, which desired nothing but pasteurized milk'. The Times, 25 October 1934. Apart from outbreaks of scarlet fever, sore throats, gastro-enteritis, a typhoid epidemic in the Bournemouth area killed 51 of the 700 affected. All these maladies were traced to infected milk. Health of the School Child, 1936 (1937), pp. 36

28. Health of the School Child, 1938 (1940),P.23. The distribution allowance for the retailer was increased from 6d. a gallon to 7d. in 1938 to encourage the small man in rural areas to join the scheme. Health of the School Child, 1937 (1938), p. 27.

29. Board of Education, Circular 1437, 5 September 1934; Circular 1443, 17 December 1935.

30. B.M.A. 'Report of Committee on Nutrition', Supplement to the British Medical Journal, 25 November 1933. For subsequent criticisms see ibid., Vol. II (1933), pp. 1132, 1144 and Vol. I (1934), pp. 36, 121, 304, 356, 774, 1006, Vol. II (1934), 1107. The figures quoted for U.A.B. benefit are the maxima. For a recalculation of the poverty line see The Times, 30 April 1938 and R.F. George, 'A new Calculation of the Poverty Line', Journal of the Royal Statistical Society c. (1937), pp. 74-95.

31. Sir J.B. Orr, Food, Health and Income (1936), pp. 21, 36, 49; C. Clark, The National Income

(1937), pp. 111-3; British Association for Labour Legislation, Report on Nutrition (1937?) summarizes the other surveys mentioned.

32. British Medical Journal, 10 April 1937.

33. B. Seebohm Rowntree, Poverty and Progress (1941), pp. 42-3, 96.

34. Health of the School Child, 1932 (1933), pp. 136, 168; Health of the School Child, 1938 (1940), pp. 21-2; Health of the School Child, 1939-45 (1947), p. 23 footnote; The Times, 13 July 1939.

35. See, for example, H. Macmillan, The Middle Way (1938), p. 308; The Next Five Years: An Essay in Political Agreement (1935), p. 199. I am indebted to Dr. D. Rolf for these references.

36. The Times, 31 March 1936. A leading article in the same issue put the case for an expansion in the provision of free and cheap milk to other members of the community. University of Birmingham Library, Chamberlain Papers, NC2/23A and NC2/24A, Chamberlain's diary, entries for 7 October 1936 and 7 February 1937. I acknowledge the permission of the Librarian of the University of Birmingham to quote from the Chamberlain Papers.

37. Hansard Fifth Series, Vol. CCCXXII, c. 200, House of Commons Debate, 7 April 1937. The rejection rate of volunteers for the army, over 50 per cent between 1923 and 1932, had been described by Lord Hankey as 'the worst deficiency' in Imperial defence; P.R.O, Ed. 24/1374, 'S. Baldwin to Lord Halifax, letter of 21 March 1934'.

38. P.R.O, Ed. 50/83, 'Conditions as regards physique, clothing, and boots of school children in S. Wales Coalfields', J.E. Underwood, 21 February 1930: his minute of 23 April 1934, his letter of 14 April 1934 to Dr. Dilys Jones.

39. British Medical Journal, Supplement, 25 November 1933; ibid., 28 December 1935.

40. R.H. Jones, 'Physical Indices and Clinical Assessment of the Nutrition of Schoolchildren', Journal of the Royal Statistical Society CI (1938), pp. 1-34.

41. Health of the School Child, 1937 (1938), pp. 21-2.

42. Health of the School Child, 1938 (1940), pp. 18-19, 22-3. P.R.O. Ed. 123/294B, 'Report of Survey, May 1939'.

43. P.H.J.H. Gosden, Education in the Second World War: A Study in Policy and Administration (1976), p. 184.

44. P.R.O, Ed. 50/214, 'Report of Survey, 1939?'.

45. P.R.O, Ed. 50/216, 'Memorandum of 16 March 1939'.

46. The Times, 9 August 1939.

47. Wartime developments are more fully discussed in P.H.J.H. Gosden, op.cit., Chapter IX.

48. P.R.O, Ed. 50/215, 'Attlee's memorandum of 7 June 1940'; 'Attlee to Ramsbotham, 12 June 1940'; 'Report of Meeting of War Cabinet Food Policy Committee, sub-heading "School Meals and Communal Feeding", 24 June 1940'.

49. P.R.O, Ed. 50/215, 'E.D. Marris's memorandum of 22 July 1941'.

50. S. Ferguson and H. Fitzgerald, Studies in the Social Services: History of the Second World War United Kingdom Civil Series (1978), pp. 156-9.

51. The Times, 1 October 1941.

52. R.J. Hammond, Food: Studies in Administration and Control, Vol. II (1951), p. 683; The Nutritional Standard of School Dinners (1965), p. 1; Nutrition in Schools (1975), p. 13.

53. R.J. Hammond, op.cit., p. 423.

54. A.J.P. Taylor, English History, 1914-45 (1965), p. 564; Health of the School Child, 1939-45 (1947), pp. 28-9.

55. P.R.O, Ed. 123/216, 'Report on a visit to Bradford, September 1943'.

56. Report of the Committee on Milk Distribution (Cmnd. 7414), p. 89.

10. THE DIETS OF THE LOCAL PRISONS 1835 TO 1878

VALERIE JOHNSTON

Because institutions were often required to keep some form of record it is, for many periods, easier to determine what types and quantities of food were consumed by inmates, such as prisoners and paupers, than it is to find out what was eaten by other sections of the population. The records of the local prison system are particularly impressive. For the years between 1835 and 1878 it is possible to find the dietary officially served in most prisons in England and Wales and in many cases the complete dietary history of an individual institution is available. It is, therefore, possible to build up a very detailed picture of the daily food-intake of prisoners and to make some analysis of the nutritional content of their diets.

The local or 'County and Borough' prisons were prisons which were administered prior to 1877 by local authorities (most frequently county justices of the peace and sheriffs or city, borough or town magistrates) as opposed to those, such as Milbank Penitentiary or the hulks, which were administered by the national government(1). There were basically three types of prison - gaols which held prisoners awaiting trial or those sentenced to very short terms, houses of correction which held prisoners who had been sentenced to longer periods and debtor's prisons - although in some instances two or even all three types of institution were contained in the same building. As debtors were allowed to bring in their own food for much of the period this study will concentrate upon the inmates of gaols and houses of correction who were more likely to have eaten only the approved prison rations.

1835 has been chosen as the starting date for this paper because it was the year in which

Inspectors of Local Prisons responsible to the
Home Secretary were first appointed and the year
in which prison rules, including the regulations
governing dietaries, became subject to certification
by the Home Secretary. In that year there were
more than 250 gaols and houses of correction
scattered throughout England and Wales(2). They
ranged in size from one room village lock-ups to
very large prisons such as the Giltspur-Street
House of Correction through which 5,000 prisoners
might pass in a year(3).

The first reports of the Inspectors(4) show
that during the 1830s the vast majority of these
prisons did make some provision for the maintenance
of prisoners. In the large gaols and houses of
correction there was usually a set dietary drawn
up by the justices, but in many of the smaller
prisons the gaoler was allowed to select rations
for the prisoners and was provided with a set sum
- often 6d. per inmate per day - to do so. Where
a prison served set dietaries female inmates often
had smaller rations than men and a house of correction might serve different diets to unemployed,
employed and hard labour prisoners. Occasionally
vagrants were given different diets from other
prisoners. Unconvicted prisoners were generally
allowed to buy part or all of their food or to
receive gifts of food from friends, although they
might lose their prison allowance if they did so.
In some prisons this privilege was shared by convicted prisoners. A few gaols and houses of correction served separate diets to prisoners doing
special work or nursing mothers. In general, however, there was no uniform system of classification,
certainly no uniform scale of rations and no national prison dietary policy.

The first standard code of practice and, indeed, the first generally accepted statement of
policy on diet was proposed by Sir James Graham,
the Home Secretary, in a report on prison discipline
published in 1843(5). Graham recommended that,
when framing a prison diet, administrators should
act on the principle that:

> The quantity of food should be given in all
> cases which is sufficient and not more than
> sufficient, to maintain health and strength,
> at the least possible cost; and that, whilst
> due care should be exercised to prevent
> extravagance or luxury in a prison, the diet
> ought not to be made an instrument

of punishment.

He went on to state that prisoners should in all cases be given three meals a day, that there should be some variety in the diet, and that all healthy adult prisoners should be dieted according to a set system of rations. Prisoners sentenced to hard labour should be given some form of animal food(6). The report contained a series of dietary tables, drawn up by the Inspectors, which were recommended for use in the prisons. These are summarized in Table 10.1. There were three diets recommended for prisoners who were not sentenced to hard labour ranging from a very scanty diety of bread and gruel for prisoners sentenced to less than a week to larger and more varied rations for those sentenced to longer terms. Five similar dietaries were proposed for hard labour prisoners. Generally, for any given term of sentence, the hard labour prisoners were to have larger portions of the main items of food than the unemployed prisoners, although there were discrepancies. Women's rations were somewhat smaller than those served to men.

The magistrates and justices of the peace who administered the county and borough prison system were not forced to accept the Graham scale of rations and, indeed, none of the diets produced by the Home Office before 1878 were mandatory. The 1843 dietaries and a slightly revised version published in 1849 were, however, fairly popular, particularly among the larger prisons, and even those local administrations which did not adopt the dietaries often made use of the Graham system of classification. By 1845, when the Eleventh Report of the Inspectors was published, 61 county and borough prisons had adopted the dietaries either in their entirety or with very slight variations(7) and the report for 1850 shows that 108 out of 185 were using the Graham rations in some form(8).

During the early 1860s there was a general swing towards increased 'deterrence' in penal policy. The Select Committee of the House of Lords which reported in 1863 favoured a policy of 'hard labour, hard fare and hard bed'(9) in the local prisons. Considerable criticism was voiced during the Committee's deliberations about the size of prison rations, particularly those served to long-term prisoners(10) and the Committee itself recommended that, while diet should continue to be sufficient, 'The low animal nature of too many

Table 10.1: Recommended Weekly Diets for Prisoners, 1843

Class(1)		Bread (oz)	Gruel (pt)	Soup (pt)	Meat (oz)	Potatoes (oz)	Cocoa (pt)
I	M and W	112	14	-	-	-	-
II	M	168	14	1(2)	-	-	-
	W	126	14	1(2)	-	-	-
III	M	168	14	2	-	-	-
	W	126	14	2	6	64	-
IV	M	168	14	3	6	64	-
	W	126	14	3	12	32	-
V	M	126	11	3	12	32	3
	W	126	11	3	16	112	3
					12	64	

(1) M – Men   W – Women

Classes

I   3 days or less
II   4-14 days
III 14 days to 6 weeks hard labour
IV   6 weeks to 3 months hard labour; over 14 days not hard labour
V   Over 3 months hard labour

(2) Hard labour only.

Source: Report Relative to the System of Prison Discipline, 1843 pp. 45.

of the criminal classes, and the admitted efficiency
of reductions in food in cases of prison offences,
render plain the value of diet as one form of penal
correction'(11). The Committee went on to recommend the appointment of a medical and scientific
commission to frame a new series of diets and in
1864 a committee of prison medical officers was
appointed by the Home Secretary. The Committee
on Dietaries of County and Borough Prisons(12)
was instructed to form dietaries that:

> should be sufficient, and not more than suffic-
> ient, in amount and quality to maintain the
> health and strength of the prisoners, and
> that the diet ought not to be in more favour-
> able contrast to the ordinary food of free
> labourers, or the inmates of workhouses, than
> sanitary conditions render necessary.

The Committee decided that diets, particularly
those of long-term prisoners, who were likely to
have committed serious offences, could safely be
made more penal if a progressive series of dietary
classes was introduced. Under the Graham system
of diets a prisoner sentenced to more than three
months was served the largest scale of rations
as soon as he entered the house of correction.
Under the proposed system a prisoner sentenced
to more than six months would start his sentence
on the lowest scale of rations - bread, potatoes
and Indian meal pudding - and would gradually progress through three more classes before achieving
the largest diet which was made up of bread, gruel,
potatoes, suet pudding, soup, cheese, and beef
after 6 months. Like the Graham rations, the 1864
Home Office diets were not mandatory and, largely
because of administrative difficulties, they never
achieved any great popularity. Many prisons continued to use the Graham diets or ration scales devised
by the justices, although a few prisons did adapt
these to the progressive system.

In 1877 the local prisons were brought under
the control of the national government and a uniform
system of prison discipline was instituted. A
new government department - the Commissioners of
Local Prisons - was appointed to administer the
system. They decided that new diets were necessary
and a new dietary committee was set up to prepare
them. The 1878 Committee on Prison Diets(13) was
told that:

In framing or recommending the dietaries for the several classes of male and female prisoners, the Committee are requested to avoid any approach to indulgence or to excess, but to arrange that the diet shall be sufficient and not more than sufficient to maintain health and strength.

In order to ensure that an element of deterrence was maintained in the diets the Committee decided to retain the practice of serving a very limited scale of rations to short-term prisoners. A modified version of the progressive system was also retained so that long-term prisoners might be seen to be punished. Under the 1878 system of classification a prisoner sentenced to more than four months would begin his term of imprisonment on the rations of the third rather than the first class and would progress to the diet of the fourth and highest class after four months.

A summary of the eight different classes of diet is shown in Table 10.2. Short-term prisoners, sentenced to less than seven days were given only bread and stirabout - a mixture of oatmeal, Indian meal and water. Men sentenced to hard labour would, after one week, be served one of a series of three diets and there was a further series of three diets for women, boys and men who were not sentenced to hard labour. As with the hard labour prisoners it was the period of sentence which determined the exact quantity of the rations. The eighth diet was intended for untried men and women. Unlike the earlier Home Office diets, the 1878 rations were mandatory and they were used in all local prisons until 1895.

In general, then, the official dietary policy of the Home Office and the Commissioners of Local Prisons was that diets in the prisons should be sufficient, but not attractive and various systems of classification were adopted to ensure that a penal element was maintained, particularly in the diets of short-term prisoners. Other means were also adopted to ensure that diets deterred or, at least, failed to attract inmates.

All prison diets were fairly circumscribed. Certain foods and drinks were usually forbidden to prisoners even in the 1830s, but more particularly after 1843. Beer very rarely appeared in a dietary, although some prison administrations allowed unconvicted prisoners to buy perhaps one half pint per day. Tea was also seldom allowed,

Table 10.2: The 1878 System of Classification

Term of imprisonment	Class of diet			
	Class I	Class II	Class III	Class IV
7 days or less	whole term	-	-	-
7 days to 1 month	7 days	remainder	-	-
1 to 4 months	-	one months	remainder	-
4 months plus	-	-	4 months	remainder

Source: Dietaries in Prisons, 1878, p. 28.

except possibly as a reward for prisoners doing
special duties or as a medical extra. Butter was
not commonly eaten in the prisons and, indeed,
the fat content of prison diets was often exceptionally low. Sugar was occasionally added to
gruel but before 1878 there were many local prisons
which made no provision for sugar at all.
Meals, on the whole, tended to lack variation.
In general between 1835 and 1878 the vast majority
of prisoners were given three meals per day. Dinner
was the largest of these and was almost always
served at midday. Breakfast and supper were usually
composed of bread served with gruel, porridge or
Indian meal pudding. Generally the same meals
were served on each day of the week, although long-
term hard labour prisoners given the Graham rations
might have cocoa three mornings a week. The most
common dinner meals were meat and potatoes, potatoes
alone, soup or suet pudding. Bread sometimes
accompanied these dishes and bread and cheese was
a fairly common meal. Dinner was not the same
on each day of the week in most instances, but
there were few prisons which served more than three
different dinner meals per week and not infrequently
only two dinners were served.
Certain rather bland and tasteless dishes
featured prominently in the dietaries of most
prisons. Gruel, made of oatmeal and water, was
one of these, as were stirabout and Indian meal
pudding which was made of maize flour and milk.
These dishes, however, were not selected only because they were unappetising. Gruel was not only
cheap but was thought to be nutritious, and any
liquid or semi-liquid food like this could be easily
prepared and served.
The foods served in the prisons and the size
of the rations changed considerably between 1835
and 1878 and it is necessary to look more closely
at the range of diets served during various periods.
The diets served at roughly twenty year intervals
- 1836, 1857 and 1878 - have been selected for
analysis. A computer programme very close to that
designed at Queen Elizabeth College, London for
studies of this type has been used to analyse the
diets. Basically it involves coding each food
in the weekly rations of the prisoners according
to tables listing the energy values and nutritional
contents of major foodstuffs taken from The Composition of Foods by R.A. McCance and E.M.Widdowson(14).
The 1836 diets are taken from the Second Report
of the Inspectors of Local Prisons(15). Bread

was definitely the most common prison food and, in most instances, it was eaten in larger quantities than other foods. Of the 153 prisons with set dietaries listed in the report there was only one - the Kendal County House of Correction(16) - in which bread was not served. The amount eaten ranged between 48½ ounces per week in a Lincoln prison to 280 ounces per week in 3 Norfolk prisons and the Pembroke House of Correction(17), but most bread rations were between 112 ounces and 224 ounces per week. Wheat flour appears to have been the most common grain used in bread, although bread composition is not often mentioned.

Gruel or porridge was served in 105 prisons. Both were generally made of oatmeal and porridge was usually, although not always, thicker than gruel and occasionally contained milk. The only other grains specifically mentioned were barley which was usually used to thicken soup and rice which was sometimes served boiled with treacle.

Potatoes were the main vegetable in the dietaries. They were served in 92 gaols and houses of correction and sometimes made up the entire dinner served to prisoners. Potatoes were almost always boiled, probably in their skins, and were often served with salt. The only other vegetables mentioned with any frequency were onions and peas. Onions were served with bread in several prisons and were often added to soup. Pea soup was also fairly common. A few other vegetables, such as leeks and carrots might also be added to soups in small amounts.

Meat (generally under one pound per week) was served in at least 79 prisons and probably, as a constituent of soup, in rather more. Beef was mentioned most frequently in recipes, but mutton was also eaten. Bacon appeared in the dietaries only occasionally. It is likely that only the cheapest cuts of meat were used - cow's head, for example, was bought to make soup. Like most prison foods, meat was usually boiled. Fish was very rarely eaten and the only type of fish mentioned in the reports was red herring.

Cheese was served in 28 prisons and it is the only solid food other than fish for which there was an obvious regional distribution. It appeared mainly in diets in prisons in agricultural counties of the south midlands and in the north of England. Milk was mentioned in the dietaries of 25 prisons, but may have been mixed with porridge or gruel in others. Like cheese, milk was seldom drunk in prisons in the central midlands or the south, although it was given to prisoners in Devon.

Beer formed a part of the normal rations of inmates in only five gaols and houses of correction, but there were other prisons in which it could be bought. Both coffee and tea were served in some of the lock-ups where prisoners were held for very short periods, but they seldom appeared in larger prisons. Prisoners in the Gloucester County Gaol and House of Correction were given hot water infused with mint to drink, but this beverage does not appear in any other dietaries(18). Salt is mentioned fairly frequently in the reports and was probably given to most prisoners gaoled for any length of time.

The differences in the forms of classification used in prisons in 1836 make it very difficult to compare diets or to obtain an average diet. There were, however, 108 prisoners for which only one main diet for men was listed. The average energy value of these diets was 2150 kcals per day, but there were many prisons with diets which were much larger or much smaller. The lowest rations were provided at the Haverfordwest County Gaol and House of Correction(19). Inmates of this prison were given 280 ounces of bread per week plus 1½ pounds of cheese and considerable amounts of gruel and pottage: a quantity of food which produced a daily energy value of over 4100 kcals. Prisoners in the small Grantham Borough Gaol and House of Correction(20) had, however, only bread and water and their energy intake was probably less than 700 kcals per day, although it is unlikely that most prisoners remained in this prison for very long.

Twenty-eight prisons (of those with diets which can be analysed) divided their inmates into two or more groups for dieting. Twelve prisons had diets for hard labour prisoners and, as might be expected, the average energy value of these diets was somewhat larger than that of the single class diets at 2510 kcals per day. Fourteen prisons had diets for inmates who did not work. The average energy value of these rations was 1980 kcals per day. A common means of differentiating between hard labour and unemployed prisoners was to give the former more meat. As a result the hard labour diets contained a greater proportion of protein and fat (13.3 per cent and 16.9 per cent) than the unemployed diets (12.2 per cent and 11.4 per cent).

216

Of the 28 prisons with dietary classifications
the Kent House of Correction in Canterbury provided
the largest rations. The Canterbury justices allowed prisoners not only bread, soup, gruel and meat
in fairly large quantities, but also provided 3
pounds of mutton per week to men doing hard
labour(21). The average daily energy value of
this diet was 3490 kcals per day, of which 36.7
per cent was derived from fat - a very large percentage in a prison diet at this time. The smallest
diet among this group was found in the Falkingham
County House of Correction(22). Bread alone was
given to vagrants who were usually sentenced to
short terms. The diet had an average daily energy
value of only 910 kcals.

Regional differences in dietary levels are
rather difficult to distinguish because of the
diverse systems of dieting, but it would appear
that, on the whole, rations in the north of England
had a higher energy value than those in the south
and that diets were larger in the west than in
the east. If a line is drawn across England to
the south of Lincolnshire and Shropshire roughly
in accordance with James Caird's map for 1850-
51(23),the average energy value of diets in counties
to the north of the line was about 2400 kcals and
in those south of the line about 2150 kcals. Sixteen of the forty prisons north of the line served
diets with an energy value of more than 2500 kcals
per day, while only 16 per cent of the prisons
south of the line had rations which came up to
this level. The main reason for the difference
in energy values between the two regions was probably the large amount of oatmeal and potatoes eaten
in the north. Both foods were also eaten in southern
England, but not in the quantities to be found
in the north, particularly in the north-west, where
oatmeal was an important working-class food. Another reason for the larger diets in the north
was that that area contained few very small prisons.
Small prisons, very numerous in southern England,
were likely to hold only those convicted prisoners
who were sentenced to short terms and, in many
cases, to have low diets which would not
have sufficed for longer periods. Finally, as
wages were higher in the north so diets were possibly higher than those of the south. Justices
of the peace may, therefore, have agreed to comparatively large rations because they thought this
was unlikely to encourage crime.

The east-west division shows less difference

in dietary levels. The English counties to the west had an average diet with an energy value of about 2310 kcals per day; those to the east about 2150 kcals. If, however, the Welsh diets are added to the survey the difference is greater. Like the northern diets, those served in the Welsh prisons tended to contain fairly large amounts of potatoes and oatmeal and, in some instances bread. As a result their average energy value was quite high. About one-third of the Welsh gaols and houses of correction had rations with an energy value of more than 2500 kcals per day.

One final regional peculiarity worth noting is the small size of dietaries in London prisons. The quantity of bread supplied on average to London prisoners was not particularly large (7 to 8½ pounds per week) and the prisons did not supply much gruel or potatoes, although some prisons provided a fairly large amount of meat. The energy value of the London diets was, therefore, quite low, although the percentage of calories derived from protein was reasonably high.

During the 1850s the publication of the Inspectors' reports became slightly erratic and some of the reports ceased to contain a description of the diets served in the majority of prisons. Fortunately, however, a return to parliament which was published in 1857(24) contains very detailed descriptions of the rations served in the most important and populous local gaols and houses of correction in every county of England and Wales. Recipes were generally included with the returns. Table 10.3 summarizes the diets of 74 prisons listed in the return and, of these, 36 used either the 1843 diets or the revised version of these diets published in 1849. The remaining prisons retained their own form of dietaries, although the majority had adopted some form of classification similar to that of the official rations. The widespread adoption of the Graham diets tended to reduce regional disparities in the types and quantities of food served. Cheese, was, for example, eaten only in Dorset, Gloucester, Hampshire and Carmarthen. Even among prisons which did not use the Graham rations there was very little variation in the composition of the diets.

The average amount of bread served to both long-term and short-term prisoners in the gaols and houses of correction which had not adopted the Graham diets was 136 ounces per week and the average amount of potatoes served to long-term

PRISON DIETS 1835-78

Table 10.3: Variety of Food in Prison Diets in the 1850s

Food

Category of Prisoners

Food	Short term (under 21 days)	Long term (more than 2 months)
Bread	38	34
Gruel	28	30
Potatoes	1	34
Soup	3	30
Meat	-	30
Porridge	6	4
Milk	2	8
Cocoa	-	5
Cheese	-	4
Irish stew	-	1
Indian-meal pudding	-	1
Suet pudding	-	4
Number of Dietaries	38	34

Source: Return of Dietaries in County Gaols, 1857

prisoners was 81 ounces per week. The size of
the meat ration, about 16 ounces per week was close
to that proposed for long-term prisoners in the
1849 Graham dietaries. The short-term diets in
prisons which had not adopted the Graham dietaries
had an average energy value of about 1520 kcals
per day, slightly greater than that of the Home
Office diets (1340 kcals per day). The long-term
diets were, however, at 2470 kcals per day, very
close in calorie content to the Class V of the
1849 version of the Graham diets (2500 kcals per
day).

Of the prisons which had not adopted the Home
Office dietaries, twenty-four had special rations
for women. The main difference between the diets
of male and female inmates lay in the quantity
rather than the quality of the food, although there
were a few prisons in which women were allowed
tea instead of gruel and special diets were given
to nursing mothers. Women in 20 prisons which
did not use the Graham dietaries were given about
120 ounces of bread per week if sentenced to terms
of one month or less. Like the men's rations this
was slightly more than the 112 ounces recommended
by the Home Office. Women sentenced to long terms
had, on average, about 108 ounces of bread per
week plus 13 ounces of meat and 68 ounces of potatoes. Both the meat and potato rations were rather
higher than those suggested by the Home Office,
but the bread ration was somewhat lower. In 13
local gaols and houses of correction definite short-
term diets (under 2 weeks) were served to women.
The average energy value of these diets was 1380
kcals per day. The lowest diet for short-term
prisoners was provided in the Gloucester Prisons
(1060 kcals), while the largest was given to prisoners in the Morpeth County Gaol (2000 kcals). There
were 12 diets designed for long-term women prisoners. The energy values of these dietaries ranged
between 1620 kcals per day in the Cambridge County
Gaol and 2500 kcals per day in the Durham County
House of Correction. On average the long-term
diets produced about 2030 kcals per day.

It can be seen from these figures that in
1857 there was still a great disparity in the size
of the diets offered by the various prisons. A
short-term diet in one prison might, for example,
be larger than a long-term diet in another. It
is very difficult, however, to put this disparity
into regional terms as the acceptance of the Graham
diets by many prisons disrupted earlier patterns.

The 1878 local prison diets are taken from the report of the Committee on Prison Diets(25). In general the foods recommended by the committee were those which were familiar to most prison administrations. Bread, stirabout, gruel, cocoa, suet pudding, potatoes and soup had all appeared in earlier dietaries. There were, however, certain innovations. Whole wheat bread was recommended and a table of substitutes which might be used to replace standard dinners was appended to the report, although it is impossible to say if and how often these substitutes were used. Among the substitutes were beans and fat bacon and fish. Prisons might also serve tinned or salt meat instead of fresh beef, although if this was done the size of the portion had to be increased. Cabbage, turnip tops, parsnips, carrots, leeks, rice and dried potatoes were also recommended as substitutes for fresh potatoes(26). On the whole the 1878 diets were rather better than the Home Office dietaries which proceeded them, but this was not true for all periods of sentence. Prisoners sentenced to less than one week had 112 ounces of bread plus stirabout.

A daily nutrient analysis of the 1878 diets is shown in Table 10.4. These rations had an energy value of about 1550 kcals per day as compared with the 1340 kcals of the 1843 diet and 1270 kcals of the 1864 short-term rations. The proportion of protein and fat in the diet was also somewhat larger in 1878.

Long-term hard labour prisoners also fared rather better. The 1878 diet for this group - 164 ounces of bread, 14 pints of porridge, 8 ounces of beef, soup, suet pudding and potatoes - had an energy value of about 2850 kcals per day. Men sentenced to long-term hard labour under the 1864 rules would have had a slightly smaller diet with an energy value of only 2660 kcals per day and would have had to pass through four smaller diets before achieving this level after six months. Men serving more than three months at hard labour on the 1843 scale would have eaten food which produced only 2190 kcals per day. The same pattern is followed generally by the women's long-term diets, although the energy value of the 1864 rations at 2280 kcals per day was slightly higher than that of the 1878 diet at 2200 kcals.

Men who were not sentenced to hard labour, however, fared rather poorly on the 1878 scale. For long terms their rations would have been the

Table 10.4: Daily Nutrient Intake of the Official Prison Dietaries, 1878

Class of Prisoner	Energy Value (kcal)	Protein (g)	Fat (g)	Carbohydrate (g)	Ca (g)	Fe (mg)
Men on Hard Labour						
I	1550	43	18	322	0.15	16.0
II	1840	56	28	361	0.20	17.0
III	2270	75	36	435	0.24	21.3
IV	2850	96	48	535	0.30	26.8
Men (Not Hard Labour) Women and Boys						
I	1550	43	18	322	0.15	16.0
II	1630	51	25	317	0.18	15.3
III	2010	69	33	379	0.22	19.2
IV	2200	71	37	425	0.23	20.8

Source: Dietaries in Prisons, 1878.

same as those given to women, while under the earlier scales they would have had rations which had
fairly high energy values - usually higher, in
fact than the hard labour diets. Some of
the interim diets - those served for periods between
one week and four months - do not compare very
favourably with the 1864 rations, but in general
most prisoners, except men who were not sentenced
to hard labour, were as well or better off than
their counterparts in 1843.

The 1878 diets were also rather better than
the average diets served in prisons which had not
adopted either the Graham rations or the 1864
dietaries. There were, however, exceptions as
a few prisons served rations somewhat larger than
any of those recommended by the Home Office or
the Commissioners of Local Prisons.

It is obvious that many of the diets served
in the local prisons between 1835 and 1878 were
inadequate. Many of the short-term diets supplied
only about half of the calories which would now
be recommended for men doing hard work and many
were also deficient in both protein and
minerals(27). In most cases these very low diets
probably did little damage as the terms for which
they were served were very short. Many prisoners
likely to be sentenced to these short terms were,
however, convicted of crimes such as drunkenness
and vagrancy for which the rate of recidivism was
fairly high. The cumulative effect of several
sentences might be serious, particularly as some
of the prisoners were probably already debilitated.
The evidence of the Rev. W.D. Morrison, Assistant
Chaplain of Wandsworth, before the 1895 Departmental
Committee on Prisons would suggest this. Morrison
stated:(28)

> There is one young fellow who came to us or
> did come to us (I suppose he is dead now)
> for short sentences, and, of course, under
> the short sentence system each time he came
> in he had to be put on the Number One diet,
> and I saw that young fellow get, what seemed
> to me, to be old very soon.

Other diets might also be deficient. Most
male prisoners sentenced to anything less than
a month were unlikely to be given rations with
an energy value of more than 2000 kcals per day
and even the long-term diets served to those sentenced to between four months and two years(29),

usually had a calorie content of less than 2700 kcals before 1878. Such diets were probably sufficient if prisoners were not required to do a great amount of work, but prison labour, particularly that termed 'Hard Labour', could be very strenuous. The tread-wheel was one of the most common forms of hard labour, but some prisons also required prisoners to turn cranks or to pick up and lower shot for long periods of time. Before 1878 the amount of labour required of hard labour prisoners varied from prison to prison, but in some houses of correction prisoners were expected to spend long periods at work(30).

> In some the treadwheel and crank are exceptional employments; in others they are universally used, but for a small part of the sentence; whilst in a third class they are the constant employments during the whole term of the imprisonment... In some they are worked for an hour without intermission; in others thirty, twenty, fifteen, ten and down to four minutes only. In some they are enforced for three hours daily, and simply as exercise; whilst in others the labour endures ten hours.

After 1878 the Commissioners recommended an ascent on the tread-wheel of 9,000 feet per day, although not for the entire duration of the sentence(31). Even rations with a calorie content of 2850 kcals per day might not have sufficed for this type of labour and the level of 2850 kcals per day was not attained under the 1878 scale until four months had been spent in prison. Moreover, some of the diets lacked more than energy. All of the government diets and many of the local authority diets for long-term inmates were deficient in calcium according to modern standards and some were deficient in protein. Most of the men's diets did contain sufficient iron. After the 1840s women were not generally required to work a tread-wheel and, as a result, they did not have to expend as much energy as men. Lack of calcium may, however, have affected pregnant women or nursing mothers. Certainly in some prisons these groups of women would have been granted special diets by the medical officer, but possibly only for short periods.

It is difficult to determine the vitamin content of the diets, but there is some evidence from medical records which indicates that prisoners did not always have sufficient vitamin C. Prisoners in the Bedford Gaol, for example, suffered in 1835 from scurvy and scurvy also appeared in several of the Essex prisons during the 1830s(32). The introduction of potatoes into most dietaries in the early 1840s reduced the incidence of scurvy in the prisons, although the disease had a brief resurgence during the potato famine(33). By 1878 the Home Office was able to report that the disease had disappeared(34).

Scurvy is the only major disease which was usually identified and was directly related to institutional diet. Most other diseases either could have been caused by other defects in prison life or might have been present before the prisoner was sentenced. Dr. Baly, the medical officer of Milbank claimed, however, that there was a connection between the rations and the incidence of tuberculosis in the prisons(35). Other surgeons blamed the type of diet and, particularly, the large amounts of oatmeal eaten, for diarrhoea, indigestion and boils(36).

Many prisoners in the nineteenth century gaol or house of correction lost weight, but loss of weight by itself need not indicate illness and there were also prisoners who gained. There is, however, some evidence from the early reports of the Inspectors that many prisoners were hungry. The Inspectors noted, for example, that in the Maidstone Gaol and House of Correction:(37)

> The work of the tread-wheel is disliked in itself, but on account of the superiority of the diet of prisoners at hard labour over that of others who do not work, the former generally considered their situation preferable. On a late occasion, when to make room for an unusual number of male convicts, the females were taken off the wheel, the latter complained that they were not fairly used, as by not working on the wheel they lost the better diet which they had whilst on it.

It is difficult to draw any real conclusions about the effect of diet upon the health of prisoners. Certainly it would seem that dietary deficiencies did cause illnesses and debilitation in the prisons of the 1830s. The official diets of 1843 and 1849 appear to have improved health standards to some extent, at least eradicating scurvy, and it is likely that health standards improved again with the 1878 scale of rations.

This study has been concerned primarily with
the dietaries of the local prisons as they were
listed in the reports of inspectors and in returns
to parliament, but it must be asked whether these
sources really describe the rations which prisoners
actually ate. The 1836 diets can be checked to
a limited extent against 'Schedule B', a form which
important prisons were required to submit each
year to the Home Secretary(38). Although many
of the diets in Schedule B do, in fact, differ
from the diets of the Inspectors' report - more,
usually, in terms of classification than food -
the foods mentioned in the two returns were similar
and the general level of the dietaries much the
same.

There is also some evidence that the Inspectors
checked the food served in prisons against the
diets returned to the Home Office, but their inspections were infrequent. It is likely that, after
the prisons came under the administration of the
Commissioners of Prisons who were known for their
regimentation of all aspects of prison life, the
rations printed in the reports were those which
were given to prisoners.

Even if it is assumed that the diets listed
in the earlier returns and reports were those
actually served in the prisons it is still question-
able whether the individual prisoner really ate
the exact rations prescribed. It is apparent from
the Inspectors' early reports that some prisons
lacked scales for weighing foods and that in others
distribution of food was left to wardsmen who were
themselves prisoners. Criticism of the methods
of distribution declined in later reports
and Mayhew's descriptions of the London prisons
of the 1850s would suggest that in these establishments, at least, some attempt was made to apportion
food correctly(39). In the event that they did
not receive the correct rations, the prisoners
had little hope of redress. A prisoner could,
in theory, demand that his rations be reweighed,
but if he exercised this right frequently he was
likely to be punished as a trouble-maker. In the
end correct distribution probably depended, before
1878, on the honesty and scrupulousness of the
warders and upon the vigilance of the prison govern-
ors and justices.

Other factors also affected the prisoner's
total food intake. Dietary punishments were very
common in gaols and houses of correction. For
an offence a prisoner might lose a meal,

be sentenced to bread and water for three days or, before 1878, be sentenced to several successive terms of bread and water. Even after 1878, when it was recommended that prisoners be given three days' normal diet between each period of punishment, punishment diets could still greatly lessen the nutritional value of the diets.

Adulteration might also lessen the value of the prisoner's rations, although it is impossible to estimate to what degree adulteration affected food quality. Most of the small prisons which existed in the first half of the century probably bought food as prisoners were admitted and from whatever source was most convenient and least expensive. Their inmates were, therefore, likely to have eaten food which was as adulterated or unadulterated as that consumed by the general public. Larger prisons usually obtained their food by contract and could check what was actually sent in to the prison against the sample submitted with tender. Whether this made any difference depended upon the vigilance exercised by the prison medical officer and the prison governor. It is likely, however, that in at least some gaols and houses of correction food was less adulterated than that sold outside. Henry Mayhew stated of the Wandsworth House of Correction that:(40)

> The butcher meat served out to prisoners, as well as potatoes, are of good quality and carefully prepared; superior to what is generally sold in many respectable eating-houses in the metropolis.

Many of the larger prisons had their own bakeries and grain was ground by prisoners in some of them so it is likely that bread, at least, was fairly pure. The 1878 Dietary Committee noted that the prisoner ate better bread than most people: 'He is not supplied with an article adulterated with alum, bone dust, chalk and other obnoxious ingredients'(41).

The way in which food was cooked did not probably diminish the nutritional content of the diet (except, perhaps, in the case of vitamins), but it might keep prisoners from eating their full rations. Unfortunately, there is little information available about the standard of cooking in gaols or houses of correction, although the Commissioners noted in 1878 that 'Very crude notions existed as to how the soup should be cooked'(42). In any case, even if well-cooked, the diets of most of the prisons both before and after 1878 were not appetising and there is some evidence that food was wasted. Gruel and stirabout seem to have been particularly disliked, especially among women prisoners(43).

Punishments, poor cooking, adulteration and unpalatable foods all tended to reduce the nutritional intake of the prisoners. Certain prisoners were, however, likely to have had more or better food than that listed in the dietaries. During the 1830s and 1840s many prisons kept their inmates in dormitories and day-rooms and appointed wardsmen to keep order. Such wardsmen usually had extra rations or were given tea or beer as a reward for their duties. The development of the separate system of prison discipline, which involved keeping prisoners apart in individual cells for the duration of their sentences, removed the need for wardsmen, but prisoners who acted as nurses in the infirmary or who had other special duties might still be rewarded. Prisoners who acted as cooks were, of course, in a position to reward themselves. The largest group of prisoners to be given an abnormal diet were, however, those who were under the care of the medical officer. The majority of these were prisoners who were ill, but pregnant women or nursing mothers or small children might also be dieted by the prison doctor. Even prisoners who lost weight or who appeared weaker than the average might be given extra rations or have their labour reduced on medical grounds. In general, however, it is likely that the majority of prisoners who were neither ill nor under punishment were served rations roughly approximate to those discussed here and that the level of diets, particularly after the mid-century, is fairly representative of actual prison rations.

NOTES

1. There were also a few prisons administered by institutions such as universities, or even by individuals, during the early part of the century; they had generally disappeared by 1850.

2. First Report of the Commissioners of Prisons Parliamentary Papers 1878 XLII, p. 36.

3. Second Report of the Inspectors of Prisons Parliamentary Papers 1837 XXXII, pp. 450-1.

4. First Report of the Inspectors of Prisons
    Parliamentary Papers 1836 XXV.
5. Report Relative to the System of Prison
    Discipline Parliamentary Paper 1843 XXV, p.
    3.
6. Ibid.
7. Eleventh Report of the Inspectors of Prisons
    - Home District Parliamentary Papers 1845
    XXI, pp. 388-435.
8. Sixteenth Report of the Inspectors of Prisons
    - Home District Parliamentary Papers 1856
    XXXII, pp. 250-263.
9. Report of the Select Committee of the House
    of Lords on the Gaols and Houses of Correction
    Parliamentary Papers 1863 IX, p. 157.
10. Ibid. For example, the evidence of Dr. Edward
    Smith, p. 109; Dr. Guy, p. 498; W. Merry,
    p. 283.
11. Ibid. p. 9.
12. Report of the Committee on Dietaries of County
    and Borough Prisons Parliamentary Papers 1864
    XLIX, p. 561.
13. Dietaries in Prisons: Report of the Committee
    on Prison Diets Parliamentary Papers 1878
    XLII, p. 55.
14. R.A. McCance and E.M. Widdowson, The Composi-
    tion of Foods (1973). A more detailed des-
    cription of the process is given in T.C.Barker,
    D.J. Oddy and J. Yudkin, The Dietary Surveys
    of Dr. Edward Smith 1862-3 (1970), pp. 35-
    8.
15. Second Report (1837) op.cit. Table 23 which
    lists the diets used in all the prisons visited
    by the Inspectors has been the main source,
    but some corrections have been made in cases
    where Table 23 differs from more detailed
    descriptions given in the body of the Report.
    Recipes are not appended to most dietaries
    so it was necessary to compile standard recipes
    based upon what directions were given.
16. Ibid. p. 496. Presumably 32 pints of gruel
    took its place.
17. Ibid. pp. 492, 494.
18. It was served in 1838 but was probably also
    drunk in 1836. See Fourth Report of the
    Inspectors of Prisons - Southern and Western
    Districts Parliamentary Papers 1839 XXII,
    p. 284.
19. Second Report (1837) op.cit. p. 494.
20. Ibid. p. 492.
21. Ibid. p. 490.

22. Ibid. p. 492.
23. J. Caird, English Agriculture in 1850-51(1852), frontispiece. The figures were obtained from county averages. In cases where a prison served several dietaries the long-term diets or the diets of convicted prisoners were used rather than those of short-term or unconvicted prisoners.
24. Return of Dietaries in County Gaols Parliamentary Papers 1857 XIV, pp. 17-143.
25. Dietaries in Prisons op.cit.
26. Ibid. p. 87.
27. For examples of modern recommended daily intakes of energy and nutrients, see P. Fisher and A.E. Bender, The Value of Food (1972), pp. 158-60.
28. Report of the Departmental Committee on Prisons Parliamentary Papers 1895 LVI, p. 480.
29. Two years was generally the longest term in a local prison. Prisoners who committed serious crimes were usually sentenced to penal servitude or transported. Penal servitude prisons were not part of the local prison system.
30. E. Smith, 'On Private and Public Dietaries', Journal of the Society of Arts, XII (1863-4), p. 218.
31. Second Report of the Commissioners of Prisons Parliamentary Papers 1878-9 XXXIV, p. 11.
32. Second Report (1837) op.cit. pp. 239, 310.
33. Committee on Dietaries, 1864 op.cit. pp. 593-4.
34. Dietaries in Prisons op.cit. p. 79.
35. W. Baly, 'On the Mortality in Prisons and the Diseases most Frequently Fatal to Prisoners', Medico-Chirurgical Transactions XXVIII (1845), p. 234.
36. Fourth Report (1839) - Southern and Western Districts op.cit. p. 363.
37. Second Report (1837) op.cit. p. 383.
38. Copies of Reports sent to the Secretary of State Parliamentary Papers 1836 XLII, pp. 3-222.
39. H. Mayhew, The Criminal Prisons of London and Scenes of Prison Life (1862).
40. Ibid. p. 518.
41. Dietaries in Prisons op.cit. p. 75.
42. Second Report of the Commissioners of Prisons op.cit. p. 75.
43. Departmental Committee on Prisons 1895 p.39.

11. THE MOVEMENT FOR PUBLIC HOUSE REFORM 1892-1914

ROBERT THORNE

In the last decades of the nineteenth century the temperance movement was successful in bringing the drink question to the front of the political stage. Such success followed the comparative failure of two earlier campaigns to produce a more sober society, the first directed at winning drinkers to the cause by moral persuasion, the second organized to secure restrictive measures through popular agitation. The tactic which had more lasting effect, at least in making drink a major issue, was that of working within the party political system. As adopted by the most outspoken of the temperance organizations, the United Kingdom Alliance, this policy did not at first imply a total commitment to one party or the other so much as a pledge of electoral support for whichever candidates were sympathetic to the movement. By the 1890s, however, its effect was to produce a polarization, with the temperance cause being incorporated in the Liberal programme while the drink interest became aligned behind the Conseratives(1).

The debate over drink and its abuse took a much narrower compass than the subject suggests for it was more concerned with the sale of drink than with its production or consumption, particularly with the sale through public houses. The innumerable bills brought before parliament towards the end of the century dealt first and foremost with the licensing system for public houses on the assumption that the control of drink outlets would be the fastest route to reform. The proposed legislation focused either on methods of licensing - whether magistrates should hold licensing authority, whether the number of licences should be limited or whether there should be some form

of popular local control - or on the powers which
the licensing system had over such matters as opening hours or the serving of children. Common to
every form of restriction, whether aiming to close
secretive back doors to pubs or to turn a whole
district dry, was the conviction that the temptations of the pub should be the first part of
the drink trade to be curtailed.

As the centre of so much attention, the pub
and its customary position in society were very
much taken for granted. The terms on which it
was criticized had been rehearsed so often that
they went largely unquestioned. As one essay put
it: 'Probably no single institution was ever so
much spoken against, or so little spoken about'(2).
Unlike other late-Victorian reform campaigns,
temperance propagandists placed little emphasis
on original social research, preferring to rely
on long-held beliefs or on their impressions of
the pub as seen from afar. Their ignorance of
the way pubs were run and who used them, as shown
by casual mistakes that their opponents were quick
to pounce on, derived from a feeling that
an institution so roundly condemned could hardly
be worth investigating(3). Equally they, like
other reformers, had become so immersed in the
means of achieving their ends that the object of
their attention was forgotten. The same was true
of the parliamentary inquiries which they helped
to instigate: each pursued the minutia of licensing
while giving only marginal attention to the part
played by the pub in the community. The selection
of evidence, and of witnesses for questioning,
did little to challenge existing assumptions.

In this context the movement for public house
reform which was initiated by the Bishop of Chester
in 1892 is especially interesting, for it had the
effect of diverting some attention at least to
questions concerning the pub which had been so
often overlooked. As a moderate temperance reform-
er he entered the debate because of a frustration
with the negative attitude of fellow campaigners:
'A merely restrictive policy, though it has done
and is doing much to control abuses and minimize
temptations, can at best serve only as a half
measure, and if pushed too far must drive
the disease inwards and provoke a mischievous reaction'(4). To close pubs could never, he thought,
eliminate drunkenness and its associated problems:
it was far better that they should be taken over
and run in such a way that any temptation

to excessive drinking was removed, to be replaced by such attractions as games, food and sober conviviality. On the same terms the pub building, rather than being turned to new use, could be transformed into a spacious and welcoming place of entertainment.

Whatever the political feasibility of such an approach, it had the advantage that it might be applied in particular places as an experiment straight away. The Bishop of Chester helped found two organizations to initiate such schemes. The examples of reformed pubs, open to anyone to visit and comment upon, brought the focus of the drink debate back to the subject of the pub itself. Whether they were a realistic alternative or not they had the effect of provoking the right kind of questions.

Public Houses

The movement for reform took hold in the midst of a period when pubs of the kind it was intended to supplant were reaching their apogee in a burst of building activity. Throughout the century there were voices to be heard complaining of the demise of traditional taverns, domestic in appearance and hospitable in atmosphere, and their replacement by vulgar public houses 'where a customer must come, like a bucket to a well, and fill himself and go away again'(5). Such transformations could be seen most often in London and the expanding cities of the Midlands and North, or in the surrounding villages which such cities swallowed up. They were part of a much wider change of scale which influenced every kind of retailing but where the drink trade was concerned the tendency to modernize and enlarge their outlets was accelerated by certain special conditions, especially the limits put on their numbers. Two kinds of restraint grew more inhibiting as the century progressed. First, ground landlords, who at one time had been happy to see pubs provided as one of the amenities on their estates, gradually grew chary of such provision and often sought to reduce the number already in existence. In Mayfair, the first Duke of Westminster reduced the forty-seven pubs and beershops he found there on his accession in 1869 to just eight 22 years later(6). Secondly, licensing magistrates became equally cautious in granting new licences and more alive to their powers in refusing the renewal of old ones. Put together the effect of both policies was to create more publess areas, especially in newly-developed suburbs, and so to force brewers and publicans to exploit the pubs they held all the more fervently. The fullest sign of such exploitation was a campaign of pub rebuilding which quite outshone anything that had gone before.

Though this transformation of pubs was in response to certain nationwide tendencies the exact pattern it followed varied from place to place. Mark Girouard has identified two campaigns in London, in 1886-92 and 1896-99, each coinciding with periods of Conservative power(7). Armed with fresh capital raised by going public, brewing companies fought to secure the best licensed properties while successful publicans speculated in the inflationary market thus created. Both brewers and publicans employed commercial architects to redesign their new acquisitions in order to maximize their potential. As far as the different sites would allow a standard architectural formula was applied; the style a brash version of the Queen Anne revival, the fittings lavish, the ornament bright and durable. Much of the necessary kit of parts - tiles, mirrors, lighting and bar furniture - came from specialist firms well-versed in the effect to be achieved. The finished product was glamorous and theatrical but what was most astonishing, at least to first-time users, was the layout of such pubs. As far as the plan was concerned the formula was intended to combine efficient service with a system of segregation to keep different classes of drinker apart. Where older pubs of the kind that were being replaced had a hierarchy of three or four rooms the new type had a central bar area from which radiated a series of small compartments, each with its own door to the street or to an internal corridor. The proliferation of compartments (sometimes reaching ten or more) was attributed to the need to provide greater privacy for customers or, at a more practical level, the need to divide the interior so that rowdyism in one part would not infect the rest. Either way, this 'typically English' system seemed to a German observer to be a graphic example of social divisiveness: 'The people that patronize such a bar...divide themselves into six distinct and different classes, and the men in one compartment would think twice before consenting to rub shoulders with the men on the other side of the partition!(8). Had they so wished temperance campaigners might have taken some of the credit for this sense of self-consciousness about drinking in public.

In Birmingham, the only other city where the pattern of rebuilding has been examined, the brewers' wish to buy and transform pubs was just as voracious and carried on after 1899 when the London campaign faded out(9). Local brewing companies, none of them with such long ancestry as their London equals, fought over a retail trade which a few years before had been dominated by independent publicans who brewed their own beer. A Home Office return of 1892 was headed by the Holt Brewery, which had gone public only five years before, owning 161 licensed properties. In second place was Mitchell's Brewery, still a private company, with 88 houses followed by Ansell's with 65 houses(10). As in London the newly-bought pubs were soon pulled down and replaced on a suitably grander scale, lavishly clothed in ceramics, glass and mirrors produced by local firms. The typical Birmingham layout was still comparatively simple: two Public Bars on the street frontage plus a Smoke Room (the equivalent of the London Saloon Bar) tucked away at the back. But the contrast to what had gone before was startling, even to the local trade journal: 'In past times improvements were generally understood to mean say the application of a few pots of paint and whitewash, a bow window and the horse-trough put upright again. But now, when a quiet-looking inn is taken in hand for alterations, the work is tremendously drastic'(11).

Throughout the country each step that the brewers took to consolidate and enhance their position compounded temperance supporters' worst fears. Whereas earlier in the century the trade had been ill-organized and fragmented, in the face of active opposition it had been forced to find a common voice and to enlarge its support by appealing to its investors and consumers. The newly-built pubs appeared to be the most blatant aspect of its campaign, encouraging existing drinkers and ensnaring new ones. Rich ornamentation outside and in seemed to flaunt their demoralizing aim and the internal divisions to encourage secret drinking amongst those who might otherwise be inhibited to enter. The compartment system, so similar to the partitions in the pawnbroker's pledge department, appeared especially contrived to promote the worst aspects of public house life - drunkenness, crime, gambling and, above all, female drinking: 'These little dens are fully patronized and it is not "Jack" in the box, but "Jill". Or, more' generally, not Jill alone, but that misguided female and her two gossips.'(12).

These though were only fresh additions to the tally of expedients supposedly used by publicans and brewers to boost their trade and like their forerunners, such as free food or harmonic meetings, their influence was never systematically studied. Whether or not the rebuilt pubs were intended to woo a new type of customer, or to develop new drinking habits, their impact was only fleetingly recorded; no more in fact than any earlier drinking places.

The common understanding of the pub, on which reformers relied as much as anyone, was still highly generalized and usually based on an outsider's view. Even at its most pretentious, in local surveys of pub use, it depended on observations made at the door or from across the street which had to take for granted the motives of those being counted. The most ambitious of such surveys was organized by W.T. Stead's Daily Paper on the Sunday after Christmas in 1903, just over a year after the well-known Daily News census of churchgoing. All the pubs in the Paddington area of London were watched throughout their opening hours by 550 enumerators who recorded the number of men, women and children customers they had but sought no other information. When set against the earlier church census, the findings represented an outright victory for Bacchus, for an average of 648 people had visited each pub. Refuting any impression that pubs were exclusively male, 22 per cent of users were women, though there was no way of telling whether they stayed to drink or fetched beer to drink at home, nor whether they came with anyone else. At least one publican in the area had established a Ladies Only Bar, with its own entrance from the street, but most women did not rely on such exclusive provision. A further 7.7 per cent of customers were children most of whom were probably fetching beer, though some may have come with their parents(13).

Two other surveys revealed a similar balance amongst pub users. Seebohm Rowntree selected three pubs in York for observation in 1900. Taken together, 25 per cent of their customers were women and 12.65 per cent children. He noted that in a respectable working-class district women were more inclined to use the jug department. Further north in Middlesbrough a census of 106 pubs and three off-licences one Sunday in 1907 showed that

each had an average of 829 customers, 23.8 per
cent of them women and 15.2 per cent children.
By contrast a third survey, made at Dewsbury in
Yorkshire, revealed a notable absence of women(14).
   The attention focused by such surveys on women
and children, or on the rivalry between drink and
religion, highlighted their intended purpose. It
bypassed questions of social class, variations
between different types of pub, and the subtle
code that distinguished who used each bar or compartment. Figures gathered in such a haphazard
and sweeping way could never be sensitive to new
initiatives by the trade or the social gradations
of the drinking public from one pub to the next.
Conscious of such ignorance, Noel Buxton and Walter
Hoare, in their contribution to C.F.G. Masterman's
The Heart of the Empire, quoted a five-fold classification of pub users:

1. The well-to-do who frequent the saloons
    of the better houses, and who may or
    may not spend more than they ought in
    drink. They are not such as would be
    dictated to as to how they should spend
    their money. In large towns this class
    is more numerous than might be expected,
    and they spend largely.
2. The City or commercial clerk, the trades-
    man, the lower middle class generally,
    who use the gilded saloons and billiard-
    rooms of the important thoroughfares
    or the respectable neighbourhood house.
3. The working class, who fill the public
    bar of the best houses and the different
    parts of medium ones.
4. The residuum, who throng the inferior
    houses and intrude themselves in the
    roughest parts of almost all.
5. The large class drawn from classes two,
    three, and four, who send for drink to
    be consumed in their houses. For this
    nearly every house has a distinct compart-
    ment(15).

Such diversity may have been unique to London -
both Buxton and Hoare were connected with East
End breweries - but in a less obvious way it might
recur anywhere that had more than one drinking
place. This view from inside highlighted some
of the complexities that, knowingly or not, the
reformers faced.

The attempt to control drinking

From its outset the temperance movement accepted the need to reinforce its exhortations by providing institutions and activities which would be as attractive and comprehensive as those associated with drink. Though inhibited by a reluctance to compete with the home life of its members, the apparatus of meetings, lectures and excursions that was established offered an alternative social world for abstainers, a chance for convivial gatherings and mutual support of the kind that any proselytizing campaign requires. From the stage of serving its own members the next obvious step was the promotion of other, less exclusive kinds of relaxation and improvement - parks and open spaces, libraries, institutes and drinkless concerts. Yet although much more open these still appealed largely to the converted, for in tone and organization they barely touched the everyday necessities of those whom it was most hoped to reach. Publicans held sway partly because they were more ready to respond to such necessities. of whatever kind. Reformers who wanted 'to see the devil cheated in his own colours' (as one of them put it) had to consider more direct forms of imitation(16).

In this respect the coffee-house movement and Working Men's Clubs both represented more realistic intentions within the temperance campaign, although in their founding support and their zealous aims they still had much in common with earlier endeavours. The idea of providing places of refreshment for workmen while away from home challenged one of the publican's obvious strengths. Pioneered in Dundee, the first English example was the British Workman Public House in Leeds, founded in 1867. From there the movement spread through the establishment of Coffee House Companies in most provincial cities and in London, linked by a central propaganda organization and a journal: in the period May 1876 - June 1879 alone, 156 companies were incorporated in England and Wales(17). Their ideal was to imitate drinking places in all but the drink - to name their premises like pubs, to use the standard fittings, or best of all to take over and use an existing pub building. As well as coffee, tea and other non-alcholic drinks they sought to offer food, entertainment, job information and overnight lodging.

Like other quasi-philanthropic enterprises,

Coffee Public Houses frequently suffered from bad management but the prediction of the trade press that they were 'a sentimental hobby' destined for an early death proved untrue in many places(18). For instance the Liverpool company, founded in 1875, had fifty-nine premises ten years later and was able to declare a 10 per cent dividend: in 1893, with five more houses, the dividend was the same(19). Yet such commercial success may have been achieved at the expense of some of the company's original ideals, for while its grander houses appealed to customers superior to those first sought, its typical premises, with minimal furnishings 'suggestive of a workhouse dining-hall', did little to encourage evening relaxation amongst the less well off. Admitting that it had failed to solve 'the problem of making the cocoa-rooms attractive as an evening resort', the Liverpool management recognized that only part of the pub's role had been replaced(20).

Although no such dovetailing was planned, the Working Men's Club movement directed its energies to filling those hours when the appeal of coffee houses was weakest(21). At the start both movements were rivals to the pub, seeking to capture workers' leisure for improving ends but, while coffee houses held true to their original resolve, clubs developed in a way that transformed their relationship to the common foe. As founder of the Working Men's Club and Institute Union, Henry Solly intended that clubs should outdo pubs in every aspect save drink for, as he said, 'all the things for which working men go to the public-house are right and good, often necessary in themselves, except much of the beer they drink there to pay for what they get'(22). Yet in order to win and keep members he was forced to let beer in: thereafter his argument was that drinking amidst the companionship of a club engendered moderation. The concession to drink heralded other gradual changes: the shift of power from patrons to members and the displacement of educational activities by amusement - outings, plays and variety concerts featuring professional performers. Solly's willingness to yield his most dogmatic principle in the end strengthened the clubs by broadening their government and extending their appeal, but on the same count they were brought closer to the institution he abhorred.

Those like Henry Solly who promoted counter-attractions to the pub assumed that their popularity would gradually destroy the strongholds of drink, painlessly creating a sober society. However, their more probable effect, like other temperance measures, was to create enclaves of virtue which left their rivals in almost as powerful a position as before. No number of dry suburban estates or drinkless taverns could outflank the customary hold of the pub in areas where it was long-established. It took more audacity to suggest the next move which was that the community should take over the drink outlets in its midst and eliminate their worst features.

The precedent for such a solution came from Scandinavia, notably from the town of Gothenburg which in 1865 entrusted the local sale of spirits to a specially constituted company. The main reason given for the transfer was the desire to remove the incentive to private profit from the trade, any surplus left after paying a 6 per cent dividend being handed over to the municipality. Similar motives influenced other aspects of the company's management: under its control the number of licences was reduced, opening hours shortened and sales to children under 18 banned. It even established reading rooms as rivals to its own outlets. This company system, to which Gothenburg gave its name, was adopted in other towns in Sweden and, after 1871, in Norway. In preference to using the net profits to reduce the rates, the Norwegian companies gave theirs to charitable purposes(23).

Among those who visited Gothenburg to see the system in action was Joseph Chamberlain, who on his return became the chief advocate of its adoption in England. In his eyes its merit was that it offered a quick means by which drink consumption and its appalling side effects could be reduced, one which the trade might find acceptable if adequate compensation was offered and furthermore which temperance organizations might support as a stepping-stone to prohibition. In keeping with his advocacy of municipal action, Chamberlain insisted that the pubs taken over should be retained and managed by local authorities rather than special trust companies, allowing each town to judge how many outlets it should have and how they should be run. Under his vigorous mayoralty Birmingham Town Council was willing to apply to drink the same treatment it had already given to gas and water supply - it voted in favour of the Gothenburg system in 1877 - but in parliament a similar measure was thrown out: the political leaders of temperance mistrusted the plan both because it would have compensated the trade and because they could not believe that local authorities were capable of running pubs in a disinterested way. Although a Select Committee reported a year later that Chamberlain's scheme deserved to be tested no legislation was passed to promote such an experiment(24).

Because no authorities adopted the Gothenburg system its practical application remained a matter for speculation: in particular, how consumption was going to be reduced and the attractions of the pub removed, and whether it would be possible for a local community to run its pubs without succumbing to the temptation to exploit their profitability. Chamberlain's proposals, though more realistic than most, were stronger on what was to be abolished than how what remained was to be managed. However in his list of possibilities was the intention that 'there would be an end to those enormous sheets of plate glass, and globe lamps, and the mirrors and the music, and the barmaids in Bloomer costume, and all that kind of thing which would disappear as by magic'(25). Clearly, under the hand of reform there would be very little to make a pub a pleasant place to linger in.

In the absence of municipal action the chance to innovate remained with the clerical and upper class reformers of the kind whose patronage helped establish coffee houses, Working Men's Clubs and other such enterprises. In the year Chamberlain's bill was rejected by Parliament, the Rev. Osbert Mordaunt, Vicar of Hampton Lucy in Warwickshire, initiated some modest changes in the village pub, which happened to be owned by the parish. The tradition already existed of the rent from the pub being used to pay the organist: Rev. Mordaunt went one step further by installing a manager on a regular salary who was allowed the profits on the sale of non-alcholic drink and food but not on the sale of beer: spirits were banned and the giving of credit forbidden. The profits from beer, in the 1890s about £30 a year, were applied to local charities including the annual harvest home and the improvement of the village water supply. Operating on so small a scale the result was no greater than the creation of a more sober parish but as a pioneering venture Hampton Lucy was referred to as 'a genuine object-lesson'. Other rural landlords who owned pubs took up the example, for instance Lord Spencer at Chapel Bampton in

Northamptonshire in 1881 and Rev. Willett at Scaynes
Hill in Sussex eleven years later(26).

Such scattered efforts by rural landowners
and clergymen received scant attention in the
continuing debate over the restriction or abolition
of licences, yet the idea they stood for lay ready
in reserve for use by those alarmed by more extreme
measures. By the time the Liberals were returned
to power in 1892 they were committed to the idea
of local veto over licences and the following year
they introduced a bill to implement that policy,
plus a similar veto over Sunday opening. In principle that seemed a genuine advance for the pro-
hibitionist cause but, as Harcourt soon realised,
temperance support for his measure was far from
united. Fast behind his proposal came an alternative bill, introduced by the Bishop of Chester
in the Lords, to allow voters to entrust the drink
trade in their district to specially established
companies. Under his scheme any new licences would
be automatically granted to such companies and
existing licences surrendered to them on payment
of proper compensation: the surplus profits after
paying a 5 per cent dividend would be given to
charitable causes(27).

Although the Bishop of Chester advocated a
company system of management in his bill similar
in character to the limited dividend companies
active in the housing field, he never totally rejected Joseph Chamberlain's plan for public ownership through local authorities. In either case
what mattered was the removal of the trade from
private ownership, the reduction of the number
of outlets, and the elimination of any profit to
the publican from sales of alcohol. Following
Rev. Osbert Mordaunt's precedent his ideal pub
would serve temperance drinks alongside beer, with
plenty of games, newspapers and other distractions.
In appearance it would be 'reasonably attractive,
not meretriciously attractive', adopting the tone
of the ordinary pub but none of its fatal
allure(28).

Though the Bishop of Chester's proposals had
the advantage, quite apart from their moderation,
of including provision for compensation, they made
no progress in parliament. A special organization
set up to lobby for them, which included Joseph
Chamberlain amongst its supporters, likewise failed,
so attention reverted once more to what might be
achieved within the existing licensing system.
The People's Refreshment House Association Ltd.

(PRHA), registered in 1896, set out to implement the Bishop's ideas on pub management wherever the opportunity might occur, following his precepts by limiting dividends and granting excess profits to public causes. To prevent the risk of takeover by the brewers each shareholder was limited to 200 £1 shares. But the Association's immediate problem, far from fighting off the brewers, was securing a foothold in a trade dominated by existing interests with little prospect of new openings. The inflationary prices at which pubs not yet owned by brewers exchanged hands in the late 1890s made it singularly difficult for outsiders to enter the stakes. Instead of bargaining for expensive freeholds, the Association sought to lease premises from sympathetic landlords which meant, in effect, that they relied on the same kind of support as the earlier experiments in reform. The first pub to be adopted, at Sparkford in Somerset, was leased from the local rector and, as at Hampton Lucy, some of its first profits were devoted to improving the village water supply. In the next two years six more pubs were leased, all but one from aristocratic owners such as the Duke of Bedford and the Hon. William Lowther. By 1900, with fourteen pubs to its name, the Association was able to vote £112 to good causes(29).

Although the initial success of the PRHA, both through its propaganda and the example it set, was not in doubt, the Bishop of Chester was willing to admit by 1900 that it was 'unfitted to deal with the field of business which is opening rapidly and widely before it'(30). He therefore welcomed imitators, especially Lord Grey's scheme for the establishment of separate trust companies to manage pubs in each county. Because the Trust House system has survived, in name if not in character, its achievement has tended to eclipse the reputation of the PRHA but throughout the Edwardian period the original reform organization and its successors worked together according to the same aims. Grey's proposal was for local companies watched over by county worthies whose standing would help ensure a sympathetic treatment by the licensing bench. One half of the companies' voting power was to be held by the directors through their possession of 20 deferred shares of £1 each. The first such company to be established was in Grey's home county of Northumberland where the magistrates lent their support by granting it a new licence in the village of Broomhill. The pub concerned, called the 'Grey Arms', opened in 1902. Its early career was spoilt by the gaoling of its first landlord for embezzlement, and subsequently a high turnover of managers, but that did not halt the progress of the company, nor of the movement as a whole(31). The Central Public House Trust Association was set up soon after the Northumberland company in 1901 in order to provide general information and advice: by 1907 it had thirty-three county-based companies affiliated to it which between them were running 233 pubs. Some of these companies had not yet paid a dividend, and their continuing weakness led to gradual amalgamations; others were eventually taken over by the PRHA; but in its early years the system of local devolution appeared to give the trusts a momentum which was only hindered by their difficulty in finding licensed premises to adopt(32).

A visitor to a reformed pub run by the PRHA or one of the Trust Companies might not recognize its peculiarities until inside the building. Since most were old pubs which had been taken over, and most were in country or small town locations, there was little to proclaim their novelty. The essential distinction was in the way they were run - the willingness of the landlord to serve food, soft drinks, tea and coffee; the availability of games indoors and out; and the sense of a much closer control over any kind of misbehaviour. The landlord's feeling of being the representative of a cause was reinforced by the incentives he was given to advance the sale of anything non-alcoholic, and the reports he had to make of any unforeseen developments. This management ethos, the crux of which was proclaimed on notices in each bar, created a slightly earnest atmosphere reminiscent of the Coffee Public Houses in their prime. Even the secretary of the PRHA admitted that his organization 'may perhaps have gone a little too far in the way of placating its principles'(33).

To fully appreciate the ideals of the reform movement it was necessary to visit a pub specially built by one of the organizations, though in the early years these were rarities. The first battle for the opportunity to build a new pub took place at Grayshott in Hampshire in 1898, three years before Lord Grey's success in Northumberland. When it became obvious that the expansion of the village there made the granting of a new licence to serve its needs highly likely, a Grayshott and District Refreshment Association was established with the

help of the PRHA. Equipped with evidence of the
beneficial effect of reformed pubs elsewhere this
Association challenged a local brewer's application
for the licence and was itself granted the provi-
sional licence that was needed before building
works could begin. Capital for the project was
subscribed by local residents and sympathizers
on the semi-philanthropic terms typical of such
projects. The pub, completed within a year, looked
quite unlike most of those being designed
for brewers at the time. On the roadside front
a large tile-hung gable projected above a ground
storey verandah giving it a character very like
the houses hidden in the hills around. Inside there
were a bar and bar-parlour much like any other
pub but in addition it had a large coffee-room
for the serving of meals and upstairs a sitting-
room, with a small library partly made up of books
given by Bernard Shaw(34). The secretary of the
association was confident that the service given
would in the same way reach a new ideal:
'The Manager is prepared to supply tea as readily
or more so than a glass of beer and at the same
price. He is a man accustomed to catering
and would never have undertaken the management
of an ordinary public house, nor would his
wife'(35).

What Reid and Macdonald, architects of the
'Fox and Pelican' at Grayshott, had provided was
a pub suggestive of quiet, domestic enjoyment,
a building which in layout and appearance echoed
the moderation of its promoters. In a sense what
they had done was to turn the clock back to create
a version of the inn or alehouse as they had been
before the transformations of the nineteenth century. It was the most recent features of pub design
that were the first to be discarded - the glittering
embellishments and small bar compartments. J.
Douglas Scott, architect of at least two Trust
Company houses, insisted that pubs should have
no small compartments 'as this encourages excessive
and secret drinking', and that any pub taken over
should have its partitions removed. His 'Kings
Arms' at Thornford in Dorset was designed to look
like a homely farmhouse, complete with an inglenook
in the bar. Only the sign distinguished what it
really was(36).

The brewers' reaction

The first reaction of the drink trade to these

reform ventures was largely dismissive. Where they appeared to be successful it was claimed that there was nothing that they were doing that brewers and publicans had not tried already, especially in the way of serving food; alternatively, when they showed signs of failing the trade was quick to suggest that commerce and philanthropy could never be mixed, least of all when the chief intention was to curb people's indulgence in the main articles being sold. The gaoling of the first manager of the 'Grey Arms' at Broomhill, or the failure of the Liverpool Public House Trust Company in running the 'Bridge Inn' at Port Sunlight, were easily relished by those long in the business(37). Yet such a cocksure attitude could only be maintained by the trade so long as it was certain of its own strength, which after the turn of the century was less and less the case.

From the euphoria of the late 1890s, when pub building activity reached its peak, the downturn in the trade's fortunes was swift, such that by 1904 the Brewers Journal reported despondently: 'Everything has been against the brewers - taxation, confiscation, general bad trade, and last, but not least, the weather'(38). It was reasonable at the time to assume that some of these misfortunes were temporary - that the sun would shine, the recent war be forgotten, and consumption pick up again - but the continued attack on the number of licensed premises was a more permanent threat which required some flexibility in handling. The immediate source of that threat was not so much at Westminster, despite a continued flow of local option proposals culminating in the Liberals' Licensing Bill of 1908, as in the renewed vigour shown by licensing benches in exercising their duties. Foremost amongst these was the Birmingham bench, which from 1894 was under the chairmanship of Arthur Chamberlain, Joseph Chamberlain's brother. He extended the practice of refusing applications for new licences, which was common enough amongst licensing benches by then, to challenging the renewal of existing licences on the grounds that they were surplus to needs. The local brewers' response was to appease his ardour by forming an organization of their own, the Birmingham Property Co. Ltd., through which compensation could be paid for the licences surrendered. About forty licences a year were given up from 1898 onwards, until 1903 when the company found itself caught between Chamberlain's increasing demands (he asked for 500 licences

to be surrendered in the following three years)
and the high compensation that had to be paid to
licence holders outside the scheme. By then
Chamberlain's high-handedness, and the inflated
statements he made at temperance meetings, exasper-
ated his fellow justices as much as they already
infuriated the trade and in 1904 he failed to be
re-elected chairman(39).

The exercise of its full discretionary powers
by the Birmingham bench was imitated elsewhere.
The Liverpool justices, under the chairmanship
of Sir Thomas Hughes, started an area by area scheme
of reduction in 1900 while in Farnham in Surrey
a year later the licensing bench treated all forty-
five licences presented for renewal as if they
were fresh applications and refused nine of
them (40). Such measures were only the most spectacular of a range of restrictions which these
and other benches imposed on the trade - the banning
of music and dancing in pubs, the closing of back
extensions, and the limitation of sales to children
- some of which were subsequently incorporated
in nationwide legislation. To this list Arthur
Chamberlain added supervisory recommendations on
the interior planning of pubs intended to make
them more open in layout and more visible to the
outside world. After his departure his successor,
Alexander F. Chance, took the argument one step
further. In 1906 he condemned the use of 'glaring
colours in terracotta', adding that 'he could not
understand why any architect should not take advantage of some of the beautiful specimens of oak buildings which they saw scattered about the country'.
'Architects', he concluded, 'ought to adopt a style
of architecture somewhat in the nature of
the surroundings of the house and its name'(41).
It was less easy to be exact in matters of style
than management but that did not mean that they
were any less important in defining the character
of a pub and its use. The reform movements had
already begun to show how design and management
might serve a common end: short of quoting their
work by name Chance indicated that he thought theirs
was the model to follow.

It is in fact a Birmingham example which has
usually been cited as evidence that the brewers
were being won round to the lessons of reform.
The 'Red Lion' at Kings Heath was completed in
1904. As if in anticipation of Chance's remarks
it was built in imitation of a fifteenth century
inn, its stone front decorated with delicate

carvings: inside, and in the garden at the back,
it had all the best modern facilities. But this
pub was only leased by the brewers Mitchells and
Butlers, not built by them, so its peculiarities
were not a direct sign of the trade's intentions:
the suburban developers who commissioned it did
more to determine its style(42). Most brewers
having overreached themselves in their building
activities of previous years were not ready, whatever the pressure, to go that far. They stuck
cautiously to experiments in serving food or other
modest improvements, and on the odd occasions they
had for building anew they seldom completely ful-
filled Chance's ideal. Yet in opinion, if not
in practice, signs of change could easily be detected. A writer in the Licensed Victuallers' Gazette,
concerned that public opinion of the trade should
be 'respectful and sympathetic', claimed that 'drink
will have to be subordinated to food and amuse-
ments', while the same newspaper a few years later
admitted that the most dazzling qualities of pub
design might be off-putting to many customers:
'The more refined citizens shudder at the fierce
display and the vulgar feel their inability to
live up to such splendour'(43). It became a common-
place to suggest that pubs should be more like
continental cafes, to which whole families could
resort without fear of stigma.

For those who were convinced that the trade
was still in peril of local option or worse, the
work of the reform organizations seemed to cry
out for more thoroughgoing imitation, for here
was an obvious means by which brewers and publicans
could demonstrate their ability to set their own
house in order. As if the way was not pointed
clearly enough already an organization sympathetic
to the trade called the True Temperance Association
was set up in 1908 to make it absolutely explicit.
Like the Bishop of Chester's first venture this
was associated with alternative legislation to
a Liberal Licensing Bill. In this case the aim
was to speed reform by removing from the justices
the power to refuse alterations to pubs where such
works were intended to improve the general accommodation; in other words to make it easier for the
trade to follow in the path of the Trust Companies
and the PRHA(44). Although its first bill failed,
the True Temperance Association returned to parliament on a number of occasions before and after
the First World War, in the meantime maintaining
its advocacy of a cause which even those it was

most keen to help did not always heed.

The impact of the First World War

Whatever further persuasion the trade needed of the efficacy of the reform idea, whether as a political gesture or not, was provided by the experience of wartime controls. The work of the Central Control Board, set up in 1915 to regulate the drink trade, has already been the subject of a number of studies all of which emphasize how its ambitions reached beyond the solving of immediate emergencies to the conduct of much wider reform experiments(45). Within a year of its establishment its orders affecting hours of sale, Sunday sales and drinking customs had been extended to cover three-quarters of the country, but not content with that the Board investigated and reported on many aspects of drink consumption and regulation: notably it gave its support to the idea of totally nationalizing the drink industry. In the light of such a proposal what was most interesting, not least to the trade, was to examine how the Board had managed the pubs in the four areas of the country where it had been allowed to purchase them as an extension of its powers of control: of these the largest were the adjoining districts of Gretna and Carlisle where 227 licensed premises and four breweries were purchased in 1916.

In its schemes the Central Control Board had two advantages which had never been available to the earlier reform organizations: it was armed with powers of compulsory purchase which allowed it to secure town centre properties as well as rural ones of the kind normally handled by reformers, and it had a monopoly within the areas concerned. Its approach could therefore be far more comprehensive, demonstrating as never before the principles which those from Joseph Chamberlain onwards had advocated. First and foremost, it closed pubs and off-licences that were regarded as unnecessary: 104 of the 227 licences had been removed by the end of 1918. Those that remained were put in the charge of managers who, following established reform practice, received a commission on the sale of food and non-alcoholic drinks. Food sales were further encouraged by being allowed at times when drink sales were not, and five of the ex-pubs were reopened as 'Food Taverns'. Though wartime limits prevented much new building these and other conversions, including the adaptation

of the old Post Office in the centre of Carlisle
to make a restaurant, gave a sense of what might
be achieved, as did a newly-built pub at Annan
which included a cinema and a bowling-green amongst
its facilities. For a regular pub-user in Carlisle
the most graphic indication of the Board's work,
apart from the limits on what could be drunk and
when and the transformation of the landlord into
a disinterested manager, was the stripping of the
pub of all its former drink associations - the
removal of the brewers' boards and advertisements,
the insertion of plain glass in the windows and
the redecoration of the interior on simple lines.
The Board's 'wholesome passion for light, cleanliness and good decorative taste' (as one reporter put it) created the same kind of well-intentioned
austerity as had characterized reformers' pubs
before the war(46).

Whether the threat of total nationalization
was real or a bluff by Lloyd George to achieve
a sense of wartime urgency, the message presented
to the brewers by the example of Carlisle
was obvious, and whatever had earlier persuaded
them to be wary of the reformers' ideals after
1919 no longer did so. The change of heart by
the trade was symbolized by two architectural
competitions organized to discover 'The Ideal Public
House', the first promoted by Allsopp and Sons
and the second by the Worshipful Company of Brewers,
both of which set terms or entrants which acknow-
ledged the new requirements of style and plan:
for instance one asked for a plan which would allow
refreshments to be served at times when alcoholic
drinks could not, while the other, in keeping with
the historicism of such projects, suggested that
the design should be 'a quiet rendering of
eighteenth-century English architecture'(47). To
similar briefs pubs throughout the country were
built, rebuilt or altered in the following years:
in the period 1922-1926 alone, 329 brewers spent
just over £12m. on such works, the results of which
were just as visible in most towns as the products
of the late Victorian building boom(48). Set back
from the road wherever possible, their Neo-Tudor
or Neo-Georgian facades spelt out the idea of the
old English inn as a place of pleasant resort:
inside, all sign of small compartments, and the
sense of furtive drinking they evoked, had been
banished in favour of open rooms in which customers
could be served seated at separate tables. In
at least one room full meals were available, for

food was now high in the trade's priorities; so
much so that a major firm of brewers, Barclay
Perkins & Co., imported a leading Trust House figure
to run their catering school(49).

The alacrity with which the trade eventually
adopted most of the principles pioneered by the
PRHA and the Trust Companies apparently left un-
resolved the dilemma of how restraint and profitability were to be combined. In one respect the
issue was avoided, for the brewers never sought
to insulate their tenants or managers from their
commercial ambitions. Although the idea of the
disinterested publican continued to be debated,
and was the subject of a Departmental Committee
investigation in 1928, its implementation got no
further. However, it was still conceivable that
if the appeal of the reformed pub had its desired
effect its customers would each spend less. If
though there were more of them that loss would
be compensated. There is some evidence that inter-
war pubs attracted a broader clientele than their
predecessors(50). Many of their features were
designed to appeal to the more respectable classes
and to women, though the evidence of earlier surveys
suggests that the latter were not as much newcomers
as often supposed. But, as half a century before,
there is more hearsay than hard fact as to who
the drinkers were. It is easier to assume that
the brewers followed the reform lead because of
political prudence rather than a refined sense
of their market, and that their innovations went
no further than necessity demanded.

NOTES

1. A.E. Dingle The Campaign for Prohibition in
    Victorian England (1980), pp. 9-10, 38-40.
    On the earlier history of the temperance move-
    ment see Brian Harrison, Drink and the Vic-
    torians. The Temperance Question in Victorian
    England 1815-1872 (1971).
2. Noel Buxton and Walter Hoare, 'Temperance
    Reform', in C.F.G. Masterman, ed., The Heart
    of the Empire (1901), p. 171.
3. For instance, the attack in the Licensing
    World, 4th January ., 1895 p. 4, on an article
    in The Woman's Signal.
4. Times, 2nd August, 1892, p. 6.
5. 'You Must Drink', All the Year Round, 18th
    June, 1864, pp. 438-9.
6. F.H.W. Sheppard (ed.), The Survey of London,

XXXIX (1977), p. 61.
7. Mark Girouard, Victorian Pubs (1975), pp. 75-77.
8. Daily Mail, 15th June, 1909, p. 6.
9. Alan Crawford and Robert Thorne, Birmingham Pubs 1890-1939 (Birmingham, 1975).
10. Parliamentary Papers, 1892 (c. 294) LXVIII, pp. 94-5.
11. Brewer and Publican, 2nd December, 1892, p. 5.
12. Daily Telegraph, 14th September, 1892, p. 3.
13. Daily Paper, 4th January, 1904, p. 3. The census also gathered information at 28 off licences but this has been excluded from the present calculations.
14. B. Seebohm Rowntree, Poverty. A Study of Town Life (1901), pp. 313-26; F.J. Marquis and S.E.F. Ogden, 'The Recreation of the Poorest', Town Planning Review, III (1912), p. 247; Dewsbury Reporter, 9th February, 1901, p.5.
15. Buxton and Hoare, op.cit., p. 172.
16. Letter from Edmund W. Holland in the Builder, 15th April, 1871, p. 277.
17. E.T. Bellhouse, 'The Coffee-House Movement', Trans. of the Manchester Statistical Society, Session 1879-80, p. 122.
18. Licensed Victuallers' Gazette, 3rd April, 1875, p. 271.
19. Coffee Public-House News, 1st July, 1885, p. 91; Caterer and Hotel-keepers Gazette, 15th March, 1893, p. 138.
20. Coffee Public-House News, loc. cit.; Porcupine, 1st November, 1879, p. 487. In his study of the Leicester Coffee and Cocoa House Company Malcolm Elliott mentions that it also acquired better-off customers than was first intended (Trans. of the Leicestershire Archaeological and Historical Society, Vol. XLVII 1971-2, p. 59).
21. The history of the club movement has been well covered in Richard N. Price, 'The Working Men's Club Movement and Victorian Social reform Ideology', Victorian Studies, Vol. XV (December 1971), pp. 117-47; John Taylor, From Self-Help to Glamour: The Working Men's Club 1860-1972 (Oxford, 1972); and Peter Bailey, Leisure and Class in Victorian England (1978), Chap. V.
22. Henry Solly, 'Working Men's Clubs and

Institutes', _Fraser's Magazine_, LXXI (March 1865), p. 390.

23. E.R.L. Gould, _Popular Control of the Liquor Traffic_ (1894); Foreign Office Commercial Reports Nos. 184 Parliamentary Papers 1890-1 LXXXIV, 274 and 279 Parliamentary Papers 1893-4 XCI.

24. James B. Brown, 'The Temperance Career of Joseph Chamberlain, 1870-1877: A Study in Political Frustration', _Albion_ IV (1972), pp. 29-44; _Report of the House of Lords Select Committee on Intemperance_ Parliamentary Papers 1878-9 (c.113) X, p. XLV.

25. Joseph Chamberlain, _Licensing Reform and Local Option_ (Birmingham, 1876), p. 21.

26. Arthur Shadwell, 'A Model Public-House and its Lessons', _National Review_, XXV (July 1895), pp. 632-5; Joseph Rowntree and Arthur Sherwell, _British 'Gothenburg' Experiments and Public-House Trusts_ (1901), pp. 9-14; Rev. Osbert Mordaunt, _Reformed Public-Houses_ (Warwick, 1898).

27. Authorized Companies (Liquor) Bill, 56 VIC.26.

28. _Times_, 2nd August, 1892, p. 6; Royal Commission on the Liquor Licensing Laws, Parliamentary Papers 1899 (c. 9075), XXXIV, Q. 69, 163.

29. Reginald Cripps, _Public-House Reform_, 2nd. edn. (1901); Rowntree and Sherwell, _op.cit._, p. 24.

30. _Times_, 3rd November, 1900, p. 8.

31. _Newcastle Daily Journal_, 28th January, 1902; Fred Topham, _Public House Trusts and Disinterested Management_ (1907), pp. 3-5.

32. Topham, _op.cit._, pp. 29-30; People's Refreshment House Association, _The PRHA Red Book_ (1926), p. 31.

33. Central Public House Trust Association, _Third Annual Report_ (1903), p. 141.

34. Rowntree and Sherwell, _op.cit._, pp. 43-49; _Caterer and Hotel-Keepers' Gazette_, 15th September, 1899, p. 421.

35. Charlotte Lyndon, Secretary of the Grayshott and District Refreshment Association Ltd., to Charles Booth, 8th September, 1899 (Charles Booth Collection, London School of Economics).

36. CPHTA, _Third Annual Report_ (1903), p. 150; _The Architect_, 14th December, 1906, p. 389.

37. _Licensed Victuallers' Gazette_, 31st July, 1903, p. 510; _Licensing World_, 28th October, 1905, pp. 299-300.

38. _Brewers' Journal_, 15th January, 1904, p. 1.

39. Arthur Chamberlain, Licensing in the City
of Birmingham: The Birmingham Surrender Scheme,
3rd edn. (Birmingham, 1903); The Birmingham
Property Co.Ltd., The Birmingham Surrender
Scheme (Birmingham, 1903).
40. Alfred T. Davies, The Licensing Problem and
Magisterial Discretion (Nottingham, 1902),
pp. 14-24.
41. Licensing World, July 21st, 1906, p. 40.
42. Building News, July 1st, 1904, pp. 73-4;
Basil Oliver, The Renaissance of the English
Public House (1947), p. 86.
43. Licensed Victuallers' Gazette, 12th April,
1906, p. 11; ibid., 8th September, 1911,
p. 8.
44. Hansard, 4th series Vol. 195, cc. 2-26 (27th
October, 1908).
45. Henry Carter, The Control of the Drink Trade
(1918); Arthur Shadwell, Drink in 1914-1922
(1923); R.M. Punnett, 'State Management of
the Liquor Trade', Public Administration,
XLIV (Summer 1966), pp. 193-211; Michael E.
Rose, 'The Success of Social Reform? The
Central Control Board (Liquor Traffic) 1915-
21', in M.R.D. Foot, (ed.) War and Society
(1973), pp. 71-84; Derek Aldcroft, 'The Control
of the Liquor Traffic in Great Britain 1914-
21', in W.H. Chaloner and Barrie M. Ratcliffe
(eds.) Trade and Transport. Essays in Economic History in Honour of T.S. Willan (Manchester, 1977), pp. 242-57; John Turner, 'State
Purchase of the Liquor Traffic in the First
World War', Historical Journal, XXIII (September 1980), pp. 589-615.
46. Birmingham Daily Post, 26th June, 1917,
p.4.
47. Brewers' Journal, 15th September, 1920, p.
390; ibid., 15th April, 1921, pp. 149-53.
48. Royal Commission on Licensing 1929-31, minutes
of evidence, p. 2137.
49. True Temperance Notes, February 1924, p. 5.
50. B. Seebohm Rowntree, Poverty and Progress
(1941), pp. 352-4.

12. RATIONING AND ECONOMIC CONSTRAINTS ON FOOD CONSUMPTION IN BRITAIN SINCE THE SECOND WORLD WAR

DOROTHY HOLLINGSWORTH

Introduction

The experience of the 1914-18 war showed how important it would be in the event of another war to plan the supplies of foods which would be available to the British people. It was very obvious that there would be shortages of shipping, labour and packing materials as well as shortage of food; that, unless controlled, prices would rise; that catering would be difficult unless advice was given on the use of new and unfamiliar foods; that campaigns to prevent waste of food must be initiated. All these and many more problems led to the development of Great Britain's wartime food policy.

In the 1914-18 war nutrition was not considered as a subject for Governmental policy until almost too late. But in 1939, the situation was fortunately very different. Between the two wars, owing both to the need which became apparent in the first world war and the growth of nutritional knowledge of all kinds - laboratory, statistical and social-interest in nutritional policy increased and many committees were set up to consider nutritional problems. The first of these, composed mainly of physiologists, was set up in 1931, 'to inquire into the facts, quantitative and qualitative, in relation to the diet of the people, and to report as to any changes therein which appear desirable in the light of modern advances in the knowledge of nutrition'. This later became the Minister of Health's Advisory Committee on Nutrition which reported in 1937(1). In 1933 the British Medical Association set up a Nutrition Committee whose terms of reference were 'to determine the minimum weekly expenditure on foodstuffs which must be incurred by families of varying size if health

255

and working capacity are to be maintained, and to construct specimen diets'(2) and, internationally, the League of Nations Mixed Committee on the Relation of Nutrition to Health, Agriculture and Economic Policy began its work(3). The findings of these committees, and also such publications as Boyd Orr's Food, Health and Income(4), produced a fund of information on which the Food (Defence Plans) Department of the Board of Trade, which was the precursor of the Ministry of Food, was able to draw in the critical years 1937-1939 during which it became increasingly clear that sound plans must be evolved. Table 12.1 shows how this conscious scientific planning in the 1939 war was to effect changes which did not occur during the 1914 war in the consumption of certain nutritionally important foods(5).

Table 12.1: Percentage changes in the consumption of certain foods in the United Kingdom during the two World Wars

Foods	1914 (percentage change from 1909-13) (%)	1943-4 (percentage change from 1934-8) (%)
Milk	-26	+28
Eggs	-40	-6
Meat	-27	-21
Vegetables	-9	+34

Source: Journal of American Dietetic Association 23 (1947).

The prewar work had indicated that, although the total supply of foods available for consumption in 1939 was adequate in respect of calories and protein, if distribution had been equitable, it was marginal in comparison with contemporary estimates of nutritional needs for calcium, vitamins A and C and thiamin, the last of these being made the more serious by the widespread prewar consumption of white flour, at that time not fortified with any nutrient, and sugar. In addition, it was known that the prewar supplies had not been equitably distributed.

Wartime changes in food supply

Table 12.2 shows the changes in estimated
supplies of foods that occurred during World War
II. The year 1946 was the first complete year
of peace and 1946-1948 were years of exceptional
difficulty - including the rationing of bread,
flour and potatoes. 1947 was the critical year.
Afterwards food supplies began to increase. The
data are derived from government statistics(6).
The table shows clearly that the changes which
occurred during the war all tended towards dullness
and lack of palatability. This trend is particularly apparent in the supplies of meat, eggs, fats,
sugar and fruit.

These changes were caused by the need to reduce
imports of food to about half their prewar weight
and to increase home production to counterbalance
this cut. The total energy supply was thus maintained at something approaching the prewar level
throughout the war by greatly increasing the home
production of such foods as potatoes and grains,
and importing foods of high energy value such as
grains, fats, dried eggs and dried milk, and boned
meat. These changes had important effects on the
food consumption habits of the whole population
and necessitated the widespread food educational
programme which was conducted by the Ministry of
Food.

The changes in the nutritional value of food
supplies are illustrated in Table 12.3 which show
that apart from total energy and fat and vitamin
A all these measures of nutritional value showed
improvement in 1946. The aggregate for 1946-1948
shows that animal protein had reverted to the prewar
value and vitamin A had just exceeded it(7). The
estimates for fat and animal protein, and their
implications, are of some historical interest.
Dietary fat can be classified under two heads,
'visible' fat, that is butter, margarine and cooking
fats and oils, and 'invisible' fat including the
cream in milk and fat in meats, fish, eggs and
grains. The total amount of fat, 'visible' and
'invisible', available per head per day before
the war was 131g. In 1940 this figure fell to
123g and by 1941 to 115g. This was one of the
worst periods of the war in Britain for
food supplies and there is some evidence that,
although bread was at that time unrationed, the
tedium of the diet was such that people were not
eating sufficient to meet their full energy require-

Table 12.2: Food Supplies after World War II as a
percentage of prewar supplies

	1946 (%)	1946-8 (%)
Milk and cheese	128	127
Meat	82	76
Fish	116	119
Eggs	92	90
Oils and fats	78	80
Sugar	79	83
Grain products	113	116
Potatoes	148	144
Other vegetables	111	114
Fruits	79	87
Tea	95	91
Coffee	117	182
Cocoa	142	133

Source: Board of Trade Journal 194 (1968).

Table 12.3: The nutritional value of food supplies
after World War II as a percentage of
prewar values

	1946 (%)	1946-8 (%)
Energy	96	97
Protein- total	111	108
animal	103	100
vegetable	121	125
Fat	86	84
Carbohydrate	102	104
Calcium	150	159
Iron	129	126
Vitamin A	95	101
Vitamin D	176	167
Thiamin	137	137
Riboflavin	114	115
Nicotinic acid	130	125
Vitamin C	112	114

Source: Board of Trade Journal 194 (1968).

ments. In the later war years the fat position improved, but at the end of 1945 and in 1946 the food supply deteriorated and only 113g fat was then available per head per day, falling in 1947 to 107g, representing 33 per cent of total energy supplies(8). This percentage was even lower than the 35 per cent which many medical authorities are now urging as a maximum for health reasons(9). There was a public outcry in 1947 over the food supply and it is probable that people were discontented partly because of the shortage of fats. At the 28th Annual Meeting of the American Dietetic Association, I said:(10)

> The amount of fat available in the diet has an important bearing on caloric consumption. When there is a shortage of fat, it follows that the bulkiness of the day's food must increase. Furthermore, without fat, other foods which may be available are rendered less palatable and may, if the stringency becomes unduly severe, actually remain uneaten. It is fairly certain, for example, that it would have been possible for the people to eat more potatoes and bread during the winter of 1940-1941 when the overall caloric position was most serious had more fat been available to eat with these 'buffer' foods.

In view of present day concern to reduce total fat consumption and to increase that of dietary fibre, this record is of interest.

As regards protein, although the total amount in the British diet throughout the war and since was and is nutritionally satisfactory, the proportion from animal sources caused anxiety during and immediately after the war. The daily supply per head varied between 37 and 44g(11), compared with about 60g in the United States and Canada, and we did not know whether that was enough. Representatives of the Ministry of Health's Advisory Committee on Nutrition and of the Committee on Nutrition of the British Medical Association had met in 1934 to try to resolve differences of opinion on this very point, which ranged from 37g to 50g 'first-class' protein daily for an adult man, and also on energy requirements(12). It was not possible to calculate accurately the consumption of animal protein by particular groups within the population from the broad averages of national statistics, but calculations based on the rations

259

and allowances of animal foods to which different categories of people were entitled could readily be made. On that basis it appeared that during the worst years 1940-41, the amount of animal protein available to an adult was about 26g a day, well below the prewar estimate of requirement. The quantities of animal protein available for children, pregnant and lactating women were thought to be adequate, though the amount available for adolescents caused concern. These facts illustrate how recent is modern knowledge about 'safe' intakes of protein. My paper to the American Dietetic Association, delivered just over 30 years ago, and officially cleared for delivery and publication, expressed our anxiety about the adequacy of the British animal protein supply for adults(13).

Rationing constraints

The Ministry of Food's job was to allocate the reduced and less attractive supplies of food more equitably than had been possible in the prewar days of much less restricted supplies. The aim of the policy was to maintain the total food supplies so as to meet the total needs of the population and at the same time to control distribution in such a way that the specific nutritional requirements of the separate categories of the population were satisfied. The policy was carried out by means of the following overall measures:

(a) Rationing animal protein foods such as meat, bacon and cheese on a more-or-less equal basis.
(b) Rationing fat on an equal basis.
(c) Rationing sugar and sweets on an equal basis.
(d) Rendering butter and margarine nutrition-ally interchangeable by adding vitamins A and D to the latter.
(e) Promoting the production, good cooking and consumption of vegetables rich in vitamins A and C.
(f) Raising the extraction rate of flour from the prewar 70 per cent to 75 per cent in the spring of 1941, to 85 per cent in March 1942 and subsequently after changes to 82½ per cent and 80 per cent in 1944, to 90 per cent in July 1946 and back to 85 per cent in

September 1946. These changes were made for supply reasons but they were made in the light of modern knowledge on the composition of the wheat grain, so that flour containing the highest possible proportion of B vitamins and the lowest possible proportion of fibre was milled. This measure, of course, also increased the iron in the diet, though not its availability. (Wartime milling techniques were deliberately designed to achieve the greatest possible concentrations of B vitamins and the least of fibre, mainly on account of bread colour. The poor absorption of iron from cereals had not at that time been observed).

(g) Improving supplies of calcium for those in greatest need of it by the distribution of milk according to physiological need; the increased consumption of milk solids, including cheese and dried skimmed milk, and the addition of calcium carbonate to flour.

(h) Leaving unrationed as long as possible an 'energy buffer' of potatoes, flour and bread. It was in fact found necessary to ration bread from 21 July 1946 until 24 July 1948 and to sell potatoes under a special control system from 9 November 1947 to 30 April 1948.

(i) Making provision for supplying unrationed meals for workers 'on the job' as an alternative to a rigid scheme of differential rations.

In addition to these measures a number of special steps were taken to protect the nutritional position of 'vulnerable groups', particularly expectant and nursing mothers, infants and children:

(a) Milk Schemes. Priority supplies of milk were available at reduced prices or free for children up to the age of 5 years and expectant mothers; priority supplies of milk were available at home at full price for other children up to the age of 18 years and nursing mothers; the Milk in Schools Scheme which was started in 1934 was considerably expanded; a milk-cocoa drink was

261

made available for adolescents in factories.

(b) School meals which drew special rations
were expanded to meet the nutritional
needs of children between 5 to 14 years
of age. Meat rations for school meals
were greater than those for industrial
canteens or ordinary restaurants.

(c) Egg Distribution. A priority supply
of eggs was made available to children
from six months to 2 years.

(d) Cod Liver Oil. An issue was made to
all expectant mothers and children up
to the age of 5 years. Expectant mothers
could obtain vitamin A & D tablets in
place of cod liver oil.

(e) Concentrated orange juice. A standardized preparation was provided for all
expectant women and children up to the
age of 5 years. Fresh oranges were
also available for children from time
to time.

(f) Special arrangements were made for certain groups of people needing special
diets, e.g. diabetics.

The rations and allocations for adults in
September 1946 are shown in Table 12.4. The measures
taken have been discussed elsewhere(14).

Some effects of rationing constraints

The results of Britain's wartime nutritional
policy can be assessed in various ways. In Britain,
detailed statistics of food consumption have been
published by the Ministry of Agriculture, Fisheries
and Food as 'Food consumption levels in the United
Kingdom' or 'Food supplies moving into consumption
in the United Kingdom' for each year since immediately before the 1939-45 war. If these food
supplies are converted into their energy value
the contributions of different groups of foods
to total energy supplies at different times can
be calculated. Tables 12.2 and 12.3 show some
of the restrictions of war(15). The government
has also made enquiries into household food consumption and expenditure almost continuously since
1941. With the help of these surveys estimates
of the food consumption of various groups of the
population - geographical groups, social groups,
households with children and others, have been

Table 12.4: Weekly rations and allowances for adults in September 1946 compared with weekly food purchases per head July-September 1976

	1946	1976
Liquid milk (pints)	2	4.75
Cheese (oz)	2	3.75
Carcass meat(1)	c.14	15.5
Corned beef(2)	2	c.4
Bacon and ham	3	4.5
Eggs (including dried eggs)	c.2	4
Butter and margarine	6	8
Cooking fats	1	2
Bread or equivalent product	c.4	c.2
Sugar	8	13
Preserves	4	2.25
Chocolate and sweets	14	n.a.
Tea	2.5	c.2.25

Note: 1. The 1946 figure is approximate as meat was rationed by money value not weight.

2. The 1976 figure is based on all canned and cooked meats.

n.a. = not available

c. = approximate values

made. Annual Reports of the National Food Survey Committee record the results of these surveys. They provide a wealth of background material for studying trends in food consumption by families(16). One of the effects of wartime control was the narrowing of the gap in consumption between the families who spend least and those who spend most on food. This was well marked for all rationed foods, but not, as would be expected, for such unrationed foods as fish and fresh vegetables. Early in the war a special study was made to compare the results of a 1938-39 survey by Murray and Rutherford(17) on milk consumption by families belonging to different food expenditure groups with that by similar families in 1943 according to the results of the National Food Survey. The results of this comparison are shown in Table 12.5. Differences in consumption of milk still existed but had been much narrowed by wartime policy.

Three further points may be made about the effects of rationing. The first relates to the artificial constraint of rationing. In the Annual Report on the National Food Survey for 1955(18) a special study was made on the effects of the removals of controls on the purchases by different types of families of different rationed foods. In the words of the official report:

> One of the most striking consequences of decontrol was the redistribution of demand for the formerly rationed foods. Until 1953-4 differences associated with family size had been compressed by the effect of rationing and the incidence of consumer subsidies. While rationing remained effective, many large families almost automatically took up their full entitlement of rationed foods and if necessary economized on other foods. This ensured that they gained maximum benefit from the subsidies, which under rationing thus acted as an important means of redistributing the national income in favour of families with children. After the end of controls, the more ample supplies available on the free market served in the main to increase the differences between households with and without children; consumption increased markedly in the latter but exhibited only slight changes in the former... In 1952, when rationing was still in full operation, differences between groups were relatively small except for cheese, for which

Table 12.5: A comparison of average weekly milk purchases between 1938-9 and 1943

Average weekly food expenditure (per head)	1938 (May-June)	1939 (May-June)	1943					
			(Feb – March)			(April – June)		
			Retail	National Scheme	Total	Retail	National Scheme	Total
(pt/h)	(pt/h)	(pt/h)	(pt/h)	(pt/h)	(pt/h)	(pt/h)	(pt/h)	(pt/h)
under 6s.11¾d.	2.3	2.2	1.84	1.21	3.05	1.81	1.38	3.19
7s.0d. to 8s.11¾d.	2.9	2.8	2.31	0.92	3.23	2.46	1.08	3.54
9s.0d. to 10s.11¾d.	3.5	3.3	2.65	0.65	3.30	3.12	0.79	3.91
11s.0d. to 12s.11¾d.	4.0	3.9	2.94	0.47	3.41	3.71	0.57	4.28
13s.0d. and over	4.9	4.0	3.33	0.25	3.58	4.28	0.33	4.61

Note: School milk has been excluded from milk supplied under the National Scheme because it was not included in the prewar survey.

Source: Murray and Rutherford; National Food Survey.

there were special entitlements, and for car-
case meat and tea, where some difference was
to be expected since children under 5 were
entitled to only half the adult ration of
meat and no tea. By 1955 the differences
had increased very markedly for all the formerly rationed foods, though not at the same
time and at different rates. The divergence
became apparent for each individual commodity
as control on it was relaxed (legally or otherwise), but the change was more marked for
butter and cooking fat than for carcass meat,
bacon and sugar...households with several
children turned from butter to margarine.
This segregation of butter-eating from mar-
garine-eating families was determined not
by social class but by the presence of children...

The second extra point refers to sweet foods.
The government did not at first foresee the pent-
up demand for chocolates and sweets. The Ministry
of Food based its estimates of likely demand for
chocolates and sweets on prewar information and
in April 1949 took these foods off the ration,
only to find the prewar demand had been smaller
than the postwar desire for sweets, and they had
to be rationed again until February 1953. This
is the only example of such a mistake made by the
Ministry of Food(19). This urgent demand for sweet
foods was a repetition of what occurred during
World War I. Vera Brittain, after her sad return
from France in the spring of 1918, recorded:(20)
'The agony of the last few weeks in France appeared
not to interest London in comparison with
the struggle to obtain sugar; the latter was discussed incessantly, but no one wanted even to hear
about the former'. When domestic sugar rationing
ended in September 1953, the ration was 12 ounces
weekly for each person. In the first quarter of
1954, the average household purchase increased
to just over 16 ounces weekly per person, and to
18 ounces by the end of the decade, after which
it slowly fell to about the quantity obtainable
on the ration in 1953.
Thirdly, each person got a fair share of what
was available and could afford to buy it. The
rations were honoured. This had an important effect
on morale.

Nutritional effects of economic constraint in the post-rationing period

Prices of food and other necessities and incomes all affect food consumption. The study made in FAO Nutrition Division in 1969 by Périssé, Sizaret and François, used information on the total food supplies of 85 countries to identify general trends of food consumption patterns as a function of income(21). Alcoholic drinks were not included in these calculations. They showed that the proportion of energy derived from fats rises steeply with income. They also showed that the proportion of energy supplied by carbohydrates, as opposed to fats, declines as income rises, ranging from 75 per cent in low income countries to 50-60 per cent or less in those with high incomes. Concealed within this trend is the switch with rising income from great dependence on starchy staple foods to increased consumption of sugar, a trend, as already discussed, that also occurred in Britain when rationing ended. On protein, they showed that all countries, irrespective of income, obtained 11-13 per cent of the energy value of their food supplies from this source, but that the proportion of the protein supply from animal sources is closely linked with income. Those income trends were noted in the Report of a Joint FAO/WHO Ad Hoc Expert Committee on Energy and Protein Requirements(22); the Expert Committee's conclusions in the trends were:

> These changes, linked with a rise in income, apparently meet consumer tastes. Nevertheless, we may rightly wonder - in face of the growing incidence of nutrition-related disorders (obesity, diabetes, cardiovascular diseases) - whether they are not, in the long run, harmful trends. It is, in any case, certainly not necessary to take the diet of the developed countries as a model of a satisfactory state of nutrition.

By comparison, the total British food supply in 1978 was equivalent to 2920 kcal (12.2 MJ) per head per day, of which 11 per cent, 40 per cent and 49 per cent were derived from protein, fat and carbohydrate respectively(23). Thus, even at the time of a falling standard of living in the United Kingdom the dietary pattern remained that of a most affluent society. A continuous rise in the consumption of alcoholic drinks led to the result that on average in 1978 the contribution from alcoholic drinks to the total food energy supply was more than half that from protein.

The results of the National Food Survey are routinely presented in terms of the proportions of the energy value of household food consumption obtained from protein, fat and carbohydrates for the various groups of households identified. The data show a pattern of increasing affluence until the early 1970s. Inflation proceeded at a faster rate in 1972 than in any of the preceding years and in that year there was a sharp rise in world food prices. Since then food prices have continued to rise and inflation has quickened. In 1972 it appeared as if the trend towards affluence in Income Group C (which contains about 40 per cent of U.K. families) had stopped but this proved to be a temporary halt. From 1967 onwards Income Group A (the richest 10 per cent of the sample) had bought more of its food energy as fat than as carbohydrate and this situation continues in a roughly steady state. It appears that any shock effect of 1972 price rises quickly wore off. For all groups of households the long term fall in the consumption of bread and flour is mainly responsible for the continuing decline in the relative contributions from carbohydrate and the compensating rise for fat.

The relative poverty of the dietary pattern for families with two adults and four or more children can be recognized from the sources of their energy supply - with 50-55 per cent from carbohydrate and 33-39 per cent from fat - and also from the deterioration in their dietary picture for protein once rationing ended. This sort of result is found whenever differences in food consumption between families with few or no children and families with many children are studied. The National Food Survey has constantly shown that the number of young dependants has a much greater influence on patterns of food consumption or nutritional adequacy of family diet than does the income of the head of the household.

Family size and age structure have this important influence for various reasons. Children eat less of most foods than do adults and have smaller requirements for energy and most nutrients. Family income, despite family allowances, does not usually increase pro rata with additional children. Baines, Leitch and Hollingsworth(24), compared the diets of

working-class families before (1937-39) and after
the war (1955-58) and showed that the addition
of a child to a family was associated with almost
no change in the family's total consumption of
fresh green vegetables and depressed consumption
of fresh fruit. Similarly, the addition of a child
hardly affected the family's total consumption
of fresh fish and was associated with depressed
consumption of processed fish and shellfish. (Fish
fingers were not available then.) Conversely,
the addition of a child was associated with greater
increases in family consumption of margarine, pre-
serves, potatoes, bread, oatmeal and oat products
and breakfast cereals - all relatively cheap foods
- than might have been expected. Liquid milk consumption was much influenced by the Welfare and
School Milk Schemes, still fully operational in
1955-58.

Consumption of all foods but milk by comparable
groups of families before and after the war was
remarkably similar, and because of government milk
schemes there was increased milk consumption in
all groups. The milk schemes, and also the government food fortification policy, contributed to
the fact that the average postwar diets of all
sizes of family were of greater average nutritional
value than their prewar counterparts. The conclusion was that 'the most important single contribution to improvement of the diet of working
class families during the past generation was the
provision of welfare foods, especially welfare
and school milk.'

Income class differences in Britain persist
but, as has been pointed out by Passmore, Hollingsworth and Robertson(25), the diets of all sections
of the community in the late 1970s were much more
uniform than they had been before the war and they
were:

of roughly the same nutritional quality. Few
people nowadays do not have a nourishing diet,
and the differences in the intakes of nutrients
between rich and poor, large and small
families, and the various regions are now
small. Furthermore, family size affects
intakes of nutrients more than does income,
but this tends largely to reflect the smaller
appetites of the children.

The most striking differences that persist are
found for fresh vegetables and fruit, eggs, fats,

sugar, potatoes, bread and other cereals. In 1978, families in income group D (income of the head of the household less than £48 a week) obtained for consumption per head about 15 per cent less than families in income group A (income of the head of the household £128 and over a week) of fresh green and other fresh vegetables, and just over half as much as fruit, but 14 per cent more eggs, 20 per cent more fats, 52 per cent more sugar, 42 per cent more potatoes, 29 per cent more cereals and over twice as much tea(26). This is a completely different picture from that reported by Barker, Oddy and Yudkin in relation to the diets of the 1860s(27). They concluded:

> ...the poorer groups in this study ate less of the cheaper and less palatable foods as well as the more palatable foods. This supports our view that people will not eat enough to satisfy their true caloric needs if the diet does not contain an adequate amount of the palatable, more, expensive foods,

a conclusion in line with the experience, already discussed, of the restrictions of the early years of World War II in Britain. The present day continuous decline in bread consumption despite the worsening economic situation is also in line with the finding of Barker et al who showed that as particular groups of workers became poorer they did not increase their consumption of bread and potatoes; they ate less of all foods.

The 1978 comparison suggests that the richer sections of the population are now taking greater heed than are the poorer sections about medical advice to moderate their consumption of eggs, fats and sugar. Their lower consumption of potatoes and cereals probably reflects a wish to avoid obesity. The richer groups of the population, particularly those living in the south-east of England, are usually the first to adopt new dietary practices - at present, moderation of diet. The National Food Survey results demonstrate the greater ease with which new and unfamiliar foods were at first taken up by the richer groups of the population; for example, shortly after dried eggs were introduced into the United Kingdom during the war the richer groups were purchasing over four times as much dried egg as the poorer groups, though they were purchasing less than twice as many shell eggs. This contrast probably results from the fact that prejudice and conservation in food habits exert a stronger influence in the poorer than in the more prosperous families. Similar differences were seen for other unfamiliar foods particularly some of those which were imported under Lease-Lend and sold under the Points Rationing Scheme. These unfamiliar foods, however, were accepted gradually by all classes and, for example, the public outcry, which arose when it was announced in January 1946 that dried egg allocations were to cease, sprang from all sections of the community(28). It will be interesting to see how long it takes the new habits of moderation to spread similarly.

In the National Food Survey the energy value of foods bought for consumption are routinely compared with the estimated energy requirements of the families surveyed; during rationing requirements were met fully. When food supplies eased and rationing ceased the average consumption rose to a maximum of an estimated 111 per cent of estimated requirements with income group A consistently above average and income group C consistently below average until 1968. After 1970, group A lost its advantage and appeared to react more strongly than group C to the effects of the economic squeeze and rising food prices.

Conclusion

The trends in food consumption in Britain since just before the Second World War have been reviewed and the influences on them of rationing restrictions and economic constraints have been discussed. The result first of rationing and more recently of economic constraints was that in 1978 there was very little difference in nutritional value between the nutritional value of the food purchases of rich and poor - for some nutrients the advantage lay with the poor. The greatest nutritional advantage of the rich appeared to rest on greater supplies of vitamin C from fruits and vegetables.

NOTES

1. Ministry of Health, First Report of the Advisory Committee on Nutrition (1937).
2. British Medical Association, Report of Committee on Nutrition (1933).
3. League of Nations, Final Report of the Mixed

Committee of the League of Nations on the Relation of Nutrition to Health, Agriculture and Economic Policy (Geneva, 1937).

4. J.B. Orr, Food Health and Income (1936).
5. D.F. Hollingsworth, 'Nutritional policies in Great Britain, 1939-46', Journal of the American Dietetic Association (23) (1947), pp. 96-100.
6. Ministry of Agriculture, Fisheries and Food, 'Food consumption levels in the United Kingdom', Board of Trade Journal 194 (1968), pp. 753-9.
7. Ibid.
8. Ibid.
9. Royal College of Physicians of London and the British Cardiac Society, 'Prevention of Coronary Heart Disease: Report of a Joint Working Party', Journal of the Royal College of Physicians of London 10, pp. 213-76.
10. Hollingsworth, 'Nutritional policies', op.cit.
11. 'Food consumption levels', op.cit.
12. Ministry of Health, Nutrition: the Report of a Conference between representatives of the Advisory Committee on Nutrition and representatives of a Committee appointed by the British Medical Association (1934).
13. Hollingsworth, 'Nutritional policies', op.cit.
14. See D.F. Hollingsworth, 'The application of the newer knowledge of nutrition' in J.C. Drummond and A. Wilbraham, The Englishman's Food (revised ed. 1957).
15. 'Food consumption levels' op.cit.
16. The series of Annual Reports of the National Food Survey Committee were published between 1955 and 1966 under the title Domestic Food Consumption and Expenditure by the Ministry of Food (1952-4) and the Ministry of Agriculture, Fisheries and Food (1955-66). Since 1967 the series is published by the Ministry of Agriculture, Fisheries and Food as Household Food Consumption and Expenditure (1967-).
17. K.A.H. Murray and R.S.G. Rutherford, Milk Consumption Habits (Oxford, 1941).
18. Ministry of Agriculture, Fisheries and Food, Domestic Food Consumption and Expenditure, 1955 (1957).
19. D.F. Hollingsworth, 'A national nutrition policy: can we devise one?' Journal of Human Nutrition 33 (1979), pp. 211-20.
20. V. Brittain, Testament of Youth (1933), p. 430.

21. J. Périssé, F. Sizaret and P. François, 'The effect of income on the structure of the diet', FAO Nutrition News letter 7, 3 (1969), p. 1.
22. United Nations, Food and Agriculture Organization/World Health Organization, Report of a joint FAO/WHO ad hoc Expert Committee on Energy and Protein Requirements WHO Technical Report Series 522 (Geneva and Rome, 1973).
23. Household Food Consumption, 1978. op.cit.
24. A.H.J. Baines, D.F. Hollingsworth and I.Leitch, 'Diets of working-class families with children before and after the second world war', Nutrition Abstracts and Reviews 33, pp. 653-68.
25. R. Passmore, D.F. Hollingsworth and J. Robertson, British Medical Journal (1979) 1, pp. 527-31.
26. Household Food Consumption 1978, op.cit.
27. T.C. Barker, D.J. Oddy and J. Yudkin, The Dietary Surveys of Dr. Edward Smith 1862-3 (1970).
28. Hollingsworth, 'Nutritional policies', op.cit.

13. MAN'S DEMAND FOR ENERGY

DEREK MILLER

This paper is about food not fuel technology. Food, measured in the basic nutritional unit, the calorie, provides energy for man and the fundamental problem facing mankind is the provision of enough energy. Hence the current obsession with the so-called world food problem: 'so-called' because many authorities now regard famine and malnutrition in the Third World as a political and socio-economic problem rather than a supply problem. Economic historians should find this relevant: certainly they are qualified to assist in its solution if only because they understand how the West dealt with similar problems in the last century.

It is important to distinguish between energy demand and energy requirement if only because the two are seldom equal. Indeed the present set of papers has stressed the importance of economic status, culture, taste and nutritional knowledge as determinants of food consumption. Of these economic status is by far the most important, and the average energy intake in rich countries is considerably more than in poor countries. Figure 13.1 shows the relationship between energy intake expressed in terms of requirements and the gross national product (GNP) for 123 countries: the correlation coefficient is 0.775 which indicates that 60 per cent of the variation of energy intake can be accounted for by economic status. The rich countries consume more than their requirements and many poor countries consume less. Intake is equal to requirement in very few countries, i.e. demand seldom equals need.

The data in Figure 13.1 are of course open to criticism. GNP is a crude estimate of economic status and energy requirements are based on

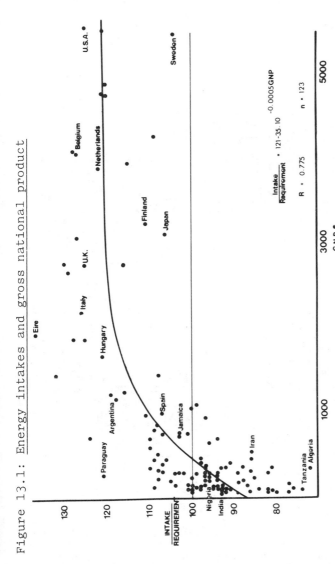

Figure 13.1: Energy intakes and gross national product

Note: Energy intakes are strictly food moving into consumption and are
expressed as a percentage of requirements.
Gross national product is expressed as US$/head/year.

Source: United Nations, Food and Agriculture Organization, Food Balance Sheets
(Rome, 1974).
O.E.C.D., Development Cooperation Review (Paris, 1974).

inadequate information. But it is clear that internationally there are wide variations in food consumption and that man displays a remarkable ability
to adapt to his food supply although the effect
of such adaptations on health is not known with
certainty. High energy intakes are associated
with various diseases of affluence and low intakes
with flagrant hunger and human misery. Nevertheless,
it is in the developing countries with poor food
supplies that population is increasing the most
and this presents a biological paradox which needs
to be resolved. It is appropriate therefore to
understand the basis of published tables of energy
requirements.

Assessment of Energy Requirements

Essentially there are three possible
approaches:

1. <u>Intake and Health risk</u> If the relationship
between intake and health were known it would be
possible to choose an optimum intake at minimum
risk. Thus low energy intakes are associated with
poor growth and high mortality whereas high intakes
are associated with obesity and heart disease.

Unfortunately these relationships are not
known with sufficient accuracy for the purpose
of assessing requirements. For example we do not
have satisfactory data on the prevalence of obesity
in Britain and morbidity data in developing
countries are worse. The measurement of food intake
of individuals is tedious and our knowledge of
food consumption especially over long periods
of time is inadequate. The development of the
diseases of affluence takes a lifetime and investigators just do not live long enough to complete
longitudinal studies. The growth of children may
be stunted by inadequate energy intakes, but high
intakes are no guarantee of fast growth. International standards for height and weight are based
on western populations on the assumption that they
are adequately fed but there is growing concern
that they are in fact overfed. Children in affluent
countries are on average bigger, i.e. both taller
and fatter, but one can question the advantages
of this. Perhaps being small really is beautiful:
certainly being slim improves longevity. The high
mortality rates of children in developing countries
are often claimed to be due to inadequate nutrition,
but the lack of sanitation must also be a factor.

Improved nutritional status does confer some resistance to infection but not universally; for example, the well nourished are more susceptible to malaria(1). In the present state of knowledge it is only possible to advise on the health risks of energy intakes below and above critical limits and then with not much certainty. For adult man these might be 1500 kcal/day and 3000 kcal/day (about 6 and 13 MJ/day), but most actual intakes fall within this range anyway.

2. Intakes of healthy populations It may be argued that healthy individuals who are neither gaining nor losing weight must be consuming enough energy to meet their needs and hence their food intake may be equated to requirements. This proposition has much to commend it, but in practice individuals are found who can maintain weight and apparent good health over a very wide range of intakes. Elsie Widdowson showed many years ago that for any 20 individuals of the same sex, age and occupation, one could be found to be eating twice that of another(2). In our own population there are some infants who customarily consume more food than some adults. Faced with data of this type, most committees on energy requirements are careful to state that their figures should only apply to the average of groups of individuals. But the mean intakes of countries (see figure 13.1) and communities show a similar variation. Recently Durnin(3) and Miller(4) have collected together survey data for communities that apparently manage to maintain weight and good health on very low intakes as shown in Table 13.1 affluent communities consume about twice these. We have recently been able to compare, by survey, communities in Ethiopia and Iran: food intakes differed by about 80 per cent, yet anthropometric measurements were almost the same in both locations. Thus again one is forced to conclude that energy requirements cannot be given as a single figure but should be expressed as a range of safe intakes. But committees setting energy requirements are reticent in providing such imprecise standards if only because they cannot be used by those responsible for food policy. Government planners require precise guidelines for organizing food supplies.

3. Measurement of energy expenditure. Energy requirements may be estimated from energy expenditure on the assumption that this represents

277

Table 13.1: <u>Communities living on low food intakes</u>

Sex	Location of survey	Energy intake (kcal/day)	(MJ/day)
Men	New Guinea	1940	8.1
	Ethiopia	1890	7.9
	Jamaica	1730	7.2
Women	USA	1770	7.4
	India	1450	6.1
	Jamaica	1440	6.0
	New Guinea	1420	5.9
	Ethiopia	1340	5.6
	USA	1330	5.6
	Puerto Rico	1240	5.2

Source: J.V.G.A. Durnin, <u>Bibliotheca Nutr. Dieta,</u>
27, p. 1; D.S. Miller, <u>Proc. Nutr. Soc.,</u>
38.

a loss that must be replaced by food. In practice this is a factorial method where the energy cost of lying at rest (the basal metabolic rate: BMR) is added to the cost of physical activity and other physiological functions. It has the advantage that individual variations particularly in physical activity may be taken into account. Much effort over the last 50 years has been devoted to measuring the energy expenditure of individuals performing various tasks, largely by indirect calorimetry, i.e. by the measurement of oxygen consumption, and a number of portable respirometers have been devised for the purpose. More recently heart rate has been used as an index of energy expenditure by means of electronic devices that record pulse rate over long periods. In addition the energy costs of growth, pregnancy and lactation have been calculated from a consideration of the energy value of the tissues synthesized and the probably efficiency of that synthetic work.

However, most measurements have been made on western populations who are in energy balance on high intakes: values for the energy expenditure for similar tasks and functions in poorly-fed populations are lower in absolute terms, although the data are more consistent if divided by body weight. This raises the dilemma of whether people should be fed according to their actual weight or what their weight would be if they were fed more food. This problem is particularly acute in the feeding of underweight children and infants who may not be able to consume recommended amounts. Raising food intakes of poor communities leads to an increase in weight in the current generation and an increase in stature in the next. The average height of Japanese that migrated to the USA increased with successive generations. Forty years ago Orr and Gilks(5) attributed the differences in adult stature between the Masai and the Kikuyu to diet rather than race and McCarrison(6) also provided data from which a similar comparison can be made between the diets of the tall Sikh and his smaller countryman the Madrassi. Coon et al., have shown the height of the genetically isolated Icelanders shrank from that of their tall Norwegian ancestors during a century of depression but returned later to make them amongst the tallest of European people(7). But even allowing for body size and differences between populations there is still much individual variation in the energy cost of performing standard tasks. Thus measurements of energy expenditure have improved the scientific basis of our understanding of the problem of energy requirements but they have not improved their precision.

FAO/WHO Energy Requirements

Because of the difficulties outlined above, most nutritionists regard tables of energy requirements with caution and some with downright scepticism: politicians and planners on the other hand treat them as gospel. Most of the committees give brief mention of health without defining it and adopt a factorial method of calculating requirement. They are all careful to point out that their figures are only to be applied to groups of individuals, an injunction which is often not followed. The latest international figures are based on a 'reference' man and woman and adjustments are made for body weight, occupation and age(8). Reference man is defined as healthy, between 20 and 40 years of age and weighing 65kg: a description of his daily life is given which is defined as moderately active. He is said to require 3000 kcal/day (12.6 MJ/day) and reference woman who is similarly described 2300 kcal/day (9.6 MJ/day). Four alternative levels of activity are also described from light to exceptionally active providing a range of requirements from 2700 to 4000 kcal for men. A table is also given to allow adjustments for body weight from 50kg to 80kg such that for moderate activity energy requirement varies from 2300 to 3680 kcal. However, the energy requirement for this group of young men (20-40 years old) can range from 2100 kcal (50kg: light activity) to 4960 kcal (80kg: exceptional activity) when both body weight and level of activity are taken into account. Allowances for declining energy expenditure with age are given: this is considered to decrease by 5 per cent for each decade between the ages of 40 to 60, and 10 per cent for each decade above 60. Additional tables list the energy requirements of infants, children, adolescents and pregnant and lactating women.

Table 13.2: Daily energy requirements

Mature weights	Developing country Males 53kg (kcal)	Females 46kg (MJ)	Developed country Males 75kg (kcal)	Females 65kg (MJ)
Child 5 years	1830	7.66	1830	7.66
Adolescent				
male	2370	9.92	3350	14.0
(14 years)				
female	2080	9.70	2780	11.6
Man	2440	10.2	3450	14.4
Woman	1840	7.70	2600	10.9

Source: FAO/WHO, WHO Tech. Rep. 522 (1973).

Using the figures in this report it is possible to calculate the energy requirements of groups of individuals in typical developing and developed countries: some sample data are shown in Table 13.2, from which it might be concluded that those from affluent countries not only consume more but actually require more. This artifact results from the importance of mature body weight in the computations and the practical difficulty of making adjustments for physical activity. Earlier FAO committees also made adjustments for climate, and since most developing countries are in the tropics this factor further emphasized the difference between the energy requirements in rich and poor countries. The present committee has rightly abandoned this concept on the grounds that man seeks thermal comfort with the use of clothes, housing, and air-conditioning: what is important is the microclimate above the skin. When the energy requirements of whole countries are calculated the differences between

rich and poor almost completely disappear because
of differences in the structure of the population
(see figure 13.2). Developing countries have young
populations with more children who require less,
whereas developed countries have more adults. Indeed
it is a useful rule of thumb to say that the average
energy requirement per head of any population is
about 2000 kcal/day or 8.4 MJ/day for every man,
woman and child.

Figure 13.2: <u>Population distribution by age and</u>
<u>average energy requirements.</u>

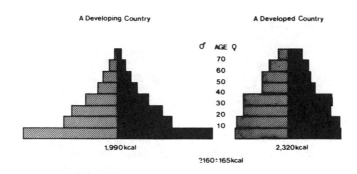

Staple Foods

A staple food may be defined as the chief
source of dietary energy. Many exist, for man
is the most omnivorous of all the animals. Human
diets may be classified according to 3 main types
of staple food, viz. cereals, vegetables, and animal
products. Figure 13.3, examples of the customary
diets of some selected countries are used
to illustrate man's opportunism in dietary adaptation: unlike other species the variety of his diet
covers the whole area of the graph. Staple foods
are as diverse as cassava in Togo, rice in Bangla-
desh, and the animal products of the Eskimo.
Whereas other species have developed by selecting
a narrow range of foods, part of man's success
must be attributed to his catholic taste: he is
the most opportunist omnivore.

There is a clear tendency for the richer
countries to consume more animal products although
these rarely reach the status of staple foods except
amongst hunting communities and specialized animal

Figure 13.3: <u>National Diets of Man</u>

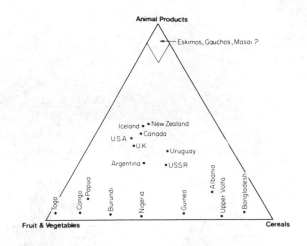

Note: The diagram is a three-dimensional graph. It shows the sources of dietary energy in selected countries. The points at each corner of the diagram represent 100 per cent of the food group indicated.

Source: FAO, <u>Food Balance Sheets</u> (Rome, 1974).

husbandrymen. This is further illustrated in Figure 13.4 which describes diets of regions classified according to their economic development. Peoples of the East are primarily cereal eaters (wheat and rice); whereas there is a tendency for those in Africa and Latin America to consume more starchy roots, tubers and fruits. With development, the old staples are increasingly replaced in favour of animal products with a greater variety of fruits and vegetables. These tendencies are true irrespective of the region or the political colour of the governments, which may indicate innate food preference for the sort of diet consumed by early man who was a hunter gatherer. It was after all only ten thousand years ago, with the development of agriculture, that nomadic peoples settled for the culture of single crops to provide them with their staple food. Great civilizations were built

Figure 13.4: Regional Diets of Man

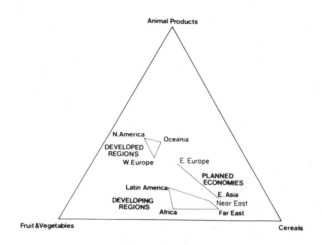

Note: The   diagram   is   a   three-dimensional   graph.
It   shows   the   sources   of   dietary   energy   in
the regions of the world.   The points at each corner
of the diagram represent 100 per cent of the food
group indicated.

Source: FAO,   Food   Balance   Sheets   (Rome,   1974).

on such dietary changes but the crops chosen were
different in different parts of the world.   Nevertheless,   the   choice   of   foods   for   the   individual
was   greatly   reduced   by   civilization   and   it   was
only when development achieved a degree of affluence
that   a   wider   variety   became   available,   although
according to Robson the choice merely represents
permutations and combinations of surprisingly few
food resources(9).   Thus looking at the world as
a whole one can perceive areas where people are
still   largely   dependent   on   single   staple   foods
and it is quite remarkable how a single species,
man, has adapted such diverse dietary ways of survival.
       The staple foods are classified in Table 13.3
according to the part of the plant consumed, e.g.
seeds, roots, tubers, fruits or stems: some indication is given where they are consumed.   The most
important group are the seeds and of these the
most important are the cereals wheat, rice and

Table 13.3: Staple Foods of the World

Food	Scientific name	Location of consumption	Origin of plant
Seeds			
Rice	*Oryza*	Far East	SE Asia
Wheat	*Triticum*	Europe, N. America	Near East
Maize	*Zea*	S. & C. America, S. & E. Africa	C. America
Sorghum	*Sorghum*	C. Africa, Far East	Africa
Bullrush millet	*Pennisetum*	N. India, S. Sahara	Africa
Finger millet	*Eleucine*	S. India, E. Africa	Africa
Foxtail millet	*Setaria*	China	China
Job's tears	*Coix*	SE Asia, Pacific	
Findi	*Digitaria*	W. Africa	
Teff	*Eragrostis*	Ethiopia	
Rye	*Secale*	Europe	Europe
Oats	*Avena*	Europe	Europe
Quinoa	*Chenopodium*	S. America	
Mongongo	*Ricinodendron*	Kalahari	
Roots and Tubers			
Irish potato	*Solanum*	Europe	S. America
Sweet potato	*Ipomoea*	S. America, Pacific	C. America
Cassava	*Manihot*	S. America, W. Africa	S. & C. America
Yam	*Dioscorea*	W. Africa, Far East	
Taro (cocoyam)	*Colocasia*	W. Africa, Pacific	SE Asia
Yautia	*Xanthosoma*	W. Africa	
Yambean tuber	*Pachyrrhizus*	S. America	
Arrowroot	*Maranta*	W. Indies	
Fruits			
Plantain	*Musa*	E. Africa	SE Asia
Breadfruit	*Artocarpus*	SE Asia, Pacific	Pacific
Jak fruit	*Artocarpus*	SE Asia	
Dates	*Phoenix*	Desert nomads	Near East
Stems			
Sago	*Metroxylon*	SE Asia, Pacific	
False banana	*Ensete*	Ethiopia	
Cycads	*Cycas*	Guam	Pacific
Bizarre			
Sugar (cane)	*Saccharum*	Sugar babies, W. Indies	Pacific
(beet)	*Beta*	Some UK children	Europe
Alcohol (grape)	*Vitis*	Some French	Near East
(barley)	*Hordeum*	Alcoholics	Near East
Fat		Some Americans	
Meat		Eskimos, gauchos	

maize, which were adopted by the great ancient civilizations in Europe, the Far East and South America respectively. Neither Caesar, the great Khans, nor the Incas could have existed without them. Nutritionally wheat has advantages over rice and maize inasmuch as it provides a greater variety of nutrients: rice diets are associated with beri-beri and maize with pellagra. Wheat and maize are milled and baked into various forms of bread which have a higher energy density than traditionally boiled rice: bread diets are less bulky. Mexican maize eaters treat their staple with alkali which renders the nicotinic acid more available, a process not adopted in the USA where there was much pellagra in the past. All three cereals are low in calcium and riboflavin, but contain enough protein to meet human needs. Thus man can almost live by bread alone, which certainly cannot be said for the starchy roots, stems and fruits. The millets and sorghums have not sustained great civilizations, but the peoples of lesser princes in Africa and India have been based on these staples. With development these and the other cereals have progressively been replaced by wheat, rice and maize, as have black rye bread by the wheaten loaf and porridge oats by cornflakes. Like rice, roots and tubers are bulky staple foods as eaten. They have the further disadvantage that they have a high moisture content and are not easily stored once harvested. However reserves may be left in the ground, and cassava is regarded by some communities as a famine staple which can be dug as required. It is a crop that is easily grown but contains virtually no protein: its high yield of energy per acre finds favour with agronomists but its lack of protein is condemned by nutritionists. The potato and the various varieties of yam and cocoyam are nutritionally superior to cassava in containing more nutrients and have certainly sustained communities in Europe, Africa and the Pacific: the potato after all was the staple food of Ireland. On a dry weight basis potatoes and yams contain almost as much protein as cereals. Most roots and tubers are simply boiled before eating but some varieties of cassava have to be elaborately washed to remove cyanide before cooking. In West Africa cassava is sometimes dried in the sun or over the fire and made into a flour, e.g. gari. Despite its disadvantages, cassava has a wide distribution and has been deliberately imported into some countries to provide food for the poor.

We even know it in Europe as tapioca.

With exception of dates, the fruit staples are starchy rather than sweet: they also have a low energy density and tend to be deficient in nutrients. The most important is the plantain, a banana used for cooking, which is the staple food of some millions of people in East Africa especially Uganda where it is made into a dough known as matoke. Breadfruit is usually eaten roasted, and is a staple food in some Pacific islands: historically it is associated with Bligh of the Bounty, who was commissioned by the British government to introduce it from Tahiti to the West Indies, but it has not found much popularity outside its original home. Dates are consumed by nomadic arabs; dried they contain 60-70 per cent sucrose plus a wide complement of nutrients. They store well and it is perhaps surprising that they are not more widely used.

The extraction of starch from the stems of palms is an elaborate and skilled art. The sago palm grows to a height of over 10 metres in about 15 years, when it is harvested. The trunk is cut up into logs, debarked, split, and the pith scooped out: the starch is then removed by washing and eventually dried. It is a staple food in parts of Malaysia, Indonesia, Thailand and the Philippines. In view of the elaborate processing one wonders how it became a staple food in the first place, especially since nutritionally it is just starch and devoid of nutrients. However, it is an island crop associated with fish consumption.

Finally, one must recognize a modern tendency for groups of people in affluent countries to have bizarre staples. With increasing wealth the consumption of highly processed foods, amounting essentially to pure chemicals, has been rising and the chief source of energy in some diets may be calculated to be items such as sugar, fat and even alcohol. Nutritionally these foods are 'empty calories' inasmuch as they are not associated with other nutrients and hence may be responsible for deficiency diseases. It is more probable that they lead to the so-called 'diseases of affluence' such as dental caries, heart disease and alcoholism.

Present Sources of Dietary Energy

The description of man's ability to adapt to a wide variety of staple foods is a fascinating academic study, but it is also a bit of a colonial tall story. Examination of primary food production data (Table 13.4) shows that the cereals, wheat, rice and maize dominate, accounting for over half the energy produced. Exotic staples hardly contribute to the total. Roots and tubers yield less than 10 per cent, and fruits only about 1 per cent. The total production amounts to 6.57×10^{18} cal per annum (GG cal/yr) which represents over 4000 kcal/head/day, i.e. enough to feed twice the present world population. However, food production is not the same as food consumption, since a large proportion of the crops produced, especially maize, is diverted to feeding livestock. World food consumption data are given in Table 13.5, from which it will be seen that the cereals, rice and wheat still dominate. Together with maize they still contribute almost half the total: roots, tubers and fruits are less than 10 per cent; sugar is now 9 per cent. Animal products account for 18 per cent including a mere 1 per cent from fish. The total energy intake is much less than the primary production but is nevertheless more than 2000 kcal/head/day and hence meets requirements at least on average. From the two sets of data, one can calculate approximately primary and secondary food production (Figure 13.5). About half of present crop production is fed to animals who then contribute less than a fifth of the food consumed by man. It is fair to ask whether this is sensible. On the credit side it may be argued that animal products are rich in nutrients; animals concentrate vitamins and minerals and provide proteins of high biological value: the ruminants also utilize foods such as forage which cannot be consumed by man. But it is extraordinary that some communities such as our own obtain more than 20 per cent of their dietary energy out of the udder of a cow. On the debit side, it must be admitted that the high consumption of animal products is to be found in affluent countries and poor countries are practically vegan. In the USA, the utilization of cereals is almost 1 tonne/head of population, mainly via animal feeding, enough to sustain six peasants in a developing country. But such statements are emotive rather than pragmatic and in the final analysis the arguments are moral or even gastronomic. Animal products are universally prized and may be regarded as a reward for economic development in both the agricultural and industrial sectors. In no way can it be claimed that affluent

Table 13.4: Primary food production of crops used
             for human consumption

	$cal/annum \times 10^{18}$	$kcal/day/hd$	% total
Wheat	1·24	849	19
Rice	1·13	774	17
Maize	1·10	754	17
Barley	0·58	397	9
Potato	0·23	158	4
Soya	0·23	158	4
Cottonseed oil	0·23	158	4
Cane sugar	0·20	137	3
Oats	0·19	130	3
Sorghum	0·18	123	3
Millets	0·16	110	2
Sweet potato	0·15	103	2
Cassava	0·15	103	2
Beet sugar	0·12	82	2
Peanuts	0·12	82	2
Rye	0·11	75	2
Coconut	0·11	75	2
Grain legumes	0·07	48	1
Sunflower seed	0·05	34	1
Grapes	0·05	34	1
Banana	0·04	27	1
Oranges	0·02	14	
Yam	0·02	14	
Etc.	0·04	27	1
Fish	0·07	48	1
TOTAL	6·57	4 514	100

Source: Derived from J.R. Harlan, 'The Plants and
         Animals that Nourish Man', Scientific
         American 235 (1976), p. 88.

Table 13.5: <u>World food consumption</u>

	kcal/hd/day	% total
Rice	507	20
Wheat	455	18
Sugar	239	9
Meat	195	8
Roots and tubers	175	7
Vegetable oils	145	6
Maize	142	6
Milk	121	5
Millets and sorghum	108	4
Animal fats	77	3
Pulses	70	3
Alcohol	62	2
Fruit	58	2
Nuts and oilseeds	52	2
Vegetables	40	2
Fish	26	1
Eggs	21	1
Etc.	70	3
TOTAL	2 563	100

Note: The data are derived from food balance sheets: hence strictly they refer to food moving into consumption.

Source: Derived from FAO, <u>Food Balance Sheets</u> (Rome, 1974).

Fig. 13.5: <u>Primary and Secondary human food production</u>

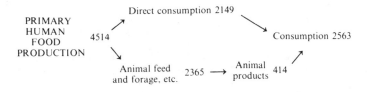

Note: The data are expressed as kcal/per person/day and are derived from Tables 13.4 and 13.5.

289

societies are robbing the poor to feed their animals since most developed countries are either self-sufficient or net exporters of food (see Table 13.6). Human consumption is a greater fraction of domestic crop production in developing countries, and those that are centrally planned are net importers.

Table 13.6: Food consumption in relation to production by area

	Consumption (human) / Primary production (domestic)
Developed countries	
Market economies	0·45
Centrally planned	0·45
Developing countries	
Africa	0·86
Latin America	0·66
Middle East	0·91
Far East	0·92
Centrally planned	1·23
World	0·48

Source: P. Levine, A. Schmitz, C. Geissler and S. Anderson, World Food Crisis in an Economic Setting (Palo Alto, 1979).

The World Food Problem

In view of the adequate crop production and adequate food consumption data presented above it is appropriate to question the nature of the world food problem. FAO have estimated the number of undernourished people in the world to be 560 millions, and it should be pointed out that this is a conservative estimate based on requirements less than their own published tables(10). Their calculations supported by clinical evidence show not only an inequitable distribution of food between nations but also within nations. Thus the world food problem is currently not a supply problem but a distribution problem: indeed it is a demand problem, because the poor cannot purchase an adequate diet. However, demographers confidently predict that the world population will double by the end of the century and hence food supplies may be in question in the future. Nevertheless, examination of past trends demonstrates that food

production has kept pace with consumption albeit
with widespread undernutrition and much of this
achievement has been attributed to the introduction
of new high-yielding varieties of cereals - the
so-called green revolution. An alternative explanation is that with economic development there has
been an increased demand for food and farmers have
responded by producing more. Pessimists point
out that in view of the obvious limits to land
area there must be limits to food production but
it can be demonstrated that these are not important
in the forseeable future. Table 13.7 shows that
the energy needs of the present population could
be met by cereal production alone on an area about
the size of the USA, or by sugar production alone
on an area about the size of Mexico. Such calculations are of course hypothetical but they do emphasize that the problem is not of land area.

Table 13.7: Man's Energy Needs and Land Area

	Yield* $cal \times 10^{-9} ha^{-1}$	Area for MEN† $sq.\ km \times 10^{-6}$	Areas of certain countries which grow the crops concerned $sq.\ km \times 10^{-6}$
Cereals alone	5 (10)	7·5 (3·6)	USA = 9·3
Roots and tubers alone	10 (15)	3·6 (2·6)	India = 3·4
Cane alone	20 (50)	1·8 (0·8)	Mexico = 2·1

Note: *Approximate average yield: the figures in
parentheses are yields currently achieved
in developed countries.
†MEN = Man's Energy Needs = 3.74 x 10^{18}
cal/year. The figures are the area of crop
required if it were the only source of food
energy for man.

Referring back, Figure 13.1 demonstrates that
those countries with a GNP greater than $1000 con-
sume more than their requirements, and these balance
the poorer countries where undernutrition is prevalent. On average the world is well fed but half
eat too much and half too little. Some countries
in both groups do better than others. The Swedes
and the Japanese apparently exercise more restraint
on their appetites than, for example, the Irish
and the Americans: the inhabitants of Eire have

the highest food consumption of all. Whether the restraint of the Swedes is due to nutrition education is not clear, but the low intakes in Japan are probably due to their bulky diet. Of the poorer countries some make better use of their meagre resources than others. For example, Paraguay has a lower GNP than Algeria but a more than adequate average intake: Algeria has the lowest food consumption of all. In a study of countries in the Far East, Quereshi (see Table 13.8) has shown that the monetary cost of meeting energy requirements from local staples is not a fixed proportion of the GNP nor is it inversely related to it as one might expect from Engel's Law, which says that the poor spend a greater proportion of income on food than the rich(11). Indonesia and Sri Lanka have a similar GNP but it takes 61 per cent of it to purchase an adequate intake in the former and only 16 per cent in the latter where there is an enlightened food policy. For the seven countries shown in Table 13.8 there is a better correlation of energy intake with the cost of food than with GNP. Further studies of this type could be of much value in food and nutrition planning.

Table 13.8: The Retail Cost of Food in Relation to Intake

Country	GNP	Cost of meeting energy requirement (% GNP)	Energy intake as a percentage of requirement
Sri Lanka	250	16	101
Thailand	380	19	105
Pakistan	170	38	99
India	150	45	93
Nepal	120	50	93
Indonesia	240	61	89
Bangladesh	110	72	—

Source: R.U. Quereshi, unpublished data.

Figure 13.1 provides no information on the changes in the compositon of the diet with increasing affluence. Quite apart from the preference for animal products, there is a marked selection in favour of energy dense foods such as sugar and fat, and against bulky diets rich in starch and fibre which retain much water as eaten. It must surely be difficult to overeat a staple food such as cooked rice or cassava which contain only one kcal/g: to meet the energy requirements it would be necessary to consume 2-3kg per day. Changes in the composition of the diet with GNP have been calculated by Périssé et al(12). They showed that energy derived from protein is constant but the relative proportions from animal and plant sources change. Energy from complex carbohydrates falls in favour of both sugar and fat with increasing GNP, and energy from both animal and vegetable fats rises. It is not clear how far these changes are inevitable. It may be that enlightened governments of developing countries will act to avoid the mistakes we have made: by so doing they might also avoid the high costs of a health service treating the various forms of overnutrition.

The Future

It is dangerous to predict, but if present trends hold mankind will continue to feed itself despite a large increase in population. One suspects that present dietary patterns will change but only slowly because of cultural conservatism: food habits are tenaciously retained even in a rapidly changing world. Hopefully energy demand will come closer to energy needs as economic development proceeds in the developing world and the affluent nations become more enlightened about the relationship between diet and health. But that may be a pious hope. Economic stagnation abroad, and the lack of food policy at home may be deciding factors in maintaining the status quo with much malnutrition and occasional famine. It seems that cereals are likely to remain the most important energy source for man and probably those isolated communities relying on curious staples will be swept aside by civilization. It is possible that new energy sources will be found which give greater yields per hectare and can be made into highly palatable dishes of good nutritional value, but present trends are not encouraging with rising consumption of sugar, fat and alcohol. Briefly the quality of energy sources is more worrying than the quantity.

Conclusion

Man's demand for food is primarily dependent upon his economic status, although this is modified by his taste, culture and nutritional knowledge.

His economic demand should not therefore be equated with his physiological needs, which depend upon body size, age, sex and physical activity. When demand and need for energy are not equal, man displays a remarkable ability to adapt to his intake, but the effect of such adaptation on health, physical performance, or reproductive ability is not known with certainty. This paper deals with the classical concepts of energy requirements but suggests that an individual can in fact maintain energy balance satisfactorily over a range of intakes. Below this range muscular wasting will occur and above it there will be and excessive deposition of fat.

Examination of the way in which energy requirements are met in practice demonstrates the wide diversity of human diets and that among animals man is the most opportunist omnivore. Most staple foods are crudely processed plant products from many species, although with economic development and affluence there is a marked preference for purified substances such as fat and sugar which are energy dense as eaten. Animal products are highly prized by most communities and provide about half the energy in the diet of rich countries. Marine products rarely contribute a significant proportion of energy intake. Man's demand for food will double in this century if only because the population will double, but the patterns of consumption are likely to remain because of cultural conservatism and economic stagnation.

NOTES

1. I.S. Dema, D.S. Miller and B.S. Platt, 'Protein metabolism in the rat with malaria', Proceedings of the Nutrition Society 18 (1959), p.xi.
2. E.M. Widdowson, 'Nutritional individuality', Proc. Nutr. Soc. 21 (1962), p. 121.
3. J.V.G.A. Durnin, 'Energy balance in man with particular reference to low intakes', Bibliotheca Nutr. Dieta 27 (1978), p. 1.
4. D.S. Miller, 'Prevalence of nutritional problems in the world', Proc. Nutr. Soc. 38 (1979).
5. J.B. Orr and J.C. Gilks 'The physique and health of two African tribes', Medical Research Council Special Report Series No. 155 (1931).
6. R. McCarrison, Nutrition and Health (1936).
7. S.C. Coon, S.M. Garn and J.B. Birdsell, Races: a Study of the Problem of Race Formation in Man (Springfield, Illinois, 1950).

294

8. United Nations, FAO/WHO, Energy and Protein Requirements WHO Tech. Rep. 522 (Geneva and Rome, 1973).
9. J.R.K. Robson, 'Changing Food habits in developing countries', Ecology of Food and Nutrition 4 (1976), p. 251.
10. Miller, 'Nutritional problems', op.cit.
11. R.U. Quereshi, personal communication.
12. J. Périssé, F. Sizaret and P. François, 'The effect of income on the structure of the diet', FAO Nutrition Newsletter 7, 3(1969), p. 1.

14. THE COST OF NUTRIENTS IN THE FIRST HALF OF THE TWENTIETH CENTURY

PAMELA MUMFORD

This study has arisen from work in devising practical diets during a period of marked change in food prices. While it is commonly believed that nutritionists are only concerned with amounts of nutrients, they are well aware that people eat foods and not nutrients, though the selection of a diet from a wide range of foods will normally satisfy nutritional requirements. Rapidly changing food prices in the 1960s and early 1970s brought to mind the fact that in the past cost was a major constraint on dietary choice. An examination of the cost of nutrients demonstrates the link between commodity prices at the farm-gate or retail level and their influence on nutrition. This interaction between cost and nutritional status is not normally perceived by historians.

If cost is the main criterion in the construction of diets it is both interesting and rewarding to identify the cheapest sources of nutrients. The economics of food and nutrition is still the most important area of nutrition to be communicated to the public, who in general have little idea of price in relation to the nutrient content of the foods they eat, and consequently are not in a position to spend limited incomes to the greatest nutritional advantage. This is in marked contrast to modern farm animal nutrition where the farmers' livelihood depends upon accurate assessment of minimum cost husbandry for maximum growth and production.

A significant feature of the British diet during the past century, and one common to all developed societies, is the increased consumption of animal products, particularly meat. Farmers have met this demand, even though foods of animal origin give lower yields both per acre and per

296

THE COST OF NUTRIENTS

man hour than plant foods and are consequently more expensive. The difference is most striking when the figures are expressed as yields of nutrients, as shown in Table 14.1. Dairy products and meats are normally regarded as good protein sources, but they provide yields per acre far lower than most of the plant sources, which as will be seen also provide greater yields of minerals and vitamins. In fact oats provide the greatest yield of calories, protein, calcium and iron per man-hour. Sugar provides the greatest energy yield per acre (6.6 Mkcal) and per man-hour (2.8 Mkcals) but contains no other nutrients. Beans compare favourably with the cereals for all nutrients, particularly protein, and are currently being promoted as an alternative protein source in both affluent and developing nations. There are certain anomalies in Table 14.1 that require comment. For example, the yields of nutrients for cabbage and carrots are greater than those for wheat flour, but the relatively low digestibility of these foods precludes their use as the sole source of nutrients: it is doubtful if the entire vitamin A potency of carrots would be available without an adequate intake of fat.

Lusk, an eminent American nutritionist, investigated the cost of nutrients in foods as long ago as the first decade of the twentieth century, and deplored the tendency of the poor to purchase prestige foods such as canned tomatoes that provided colour and flavour in a dilute watery solution - this was before the discovery of vitamin C and plant precursors of vitamin A. He was mainly concerned with cheap energy sources, which he found to be glucose, cornmeal, wheat flour, oatmeal, cane sugar, dried beans, lard, rice, bread, margarine, potatoes and butter, in that order.

The cost of nutrients in British foods was examined in March 1965, January 1974 and June 1975, during which period there was rapid inflation and additional food price changes followed when Britain joined the European Economic Community(1). The surveys were carried out in London supermarkets and high street shops in the southeast, northern and southwestern districts, and in a number of large street markets. The prices used in these calculations are the lowest that could be found, taking advantage of cut-price offers, discounts and quantity buying; for example purchasing 3lb bags of flour rather than 1 lb. Of course the housewife may not have time to shop around, and

Table 14.1: Annual yield of nutrients per acre (a) and per 100 man-hours of labour (b)

	Calories (Mkcals)		Protein (kg)		Calcium (kg)		Iron (kg)		Vitamin A (M i.u.)		Vitamin C (kg)	
	a	b	a	b	a	b	a	b	a	b	a	b
Dairy products	0.2	0.7	10	27	0.3	0.8	0	0	1	2	0	0
Chicken and eggs	0.1	0.3	12	27	0.1	0.1	0	0	1	1	0	0
Pigs	0.5	1.6	8	27	0	0	0	0	0	0	0	0
Beef	0.1	0.3	4	18	0	0	0	0	0	0	0	0
Lamb	0.1	0.5	6	27	0	0	0	0	0	0	0	0
Flour, white	0.8	9.3	27	280	0.2	0.4	2	26	0	0	0	0
Oats	1.0	11.0	36	395	0.2	2.2	13	144	0	0	0	0
Potatoes	2.3	3.4	54	77	0.4	0.5	20	29	1	2	0.3	0.4
Beans, dry	1.1	4.2	68	263	0.5	1.8	32	122	0	0	0	0
Cabbage	0.9	0.8	45	40	1.5	1.3	16	15	5	5	1.7	1.6
Carrots	2.7	0.8	77	23	2.4	0.7	48	15	431	133	0.4	0.1
Tomatoes	0.4	0.2	19	10	0.2	0.1	11	6	24	14	0.5	0.3
Apples	1.1	0.9	6	5	0.1	0.1	5	4	1	1	0.1	0.1

O indicates that the yield of nutrient expressed in this way is insignificant, though not necessarily entirely absent.

possible savings in the shopping basket may also
be offset by the cost of travel to the shops.
However, it appeared that the food bill could be
reduced by about 20 per cent with careful shopping,
and possibly even more if advantage was taken of
bulk buying. The same methodology was used for
each set of calculations. Energy content and five
of the nutrients essential to man were chosen as
key indicators of the nutritive value of the selected foods - calories, protein, calcium, iron, vitamins A and C. Nutritionists are far from unanimous
in their assessment of nutrient intakes necessary
for the maintenance of optimum health, and the
recommended intakes quoted in the column headings
of Table 14.2 are composite figures derived from
the publications of the United Nations' Food and
Agriculture Organization (FAO) and World Health
Organization (WHO), and the United Kingdom's Department of Health and Social Security (DHSS).
Recommended intakes of nutrients vary according
to age, sex, activity and physiological state of
the individual, e.g. pregnancy and lactation, and
figures used in Table 14.2 are the average for
adult men and women of sedentary occupation. Generally, where the two authorities disagree, the
lower figure has been adopted. Thus for energy,
a figure of 2500 kcals/day was taken. This is
an average of the DHSS figures for sedentary men
(2700 kcals/day) and women (2200 kcals/day), which
are set relatively low because of concern about
the high prevalence of obesity in the population.
      Protein was the other major nutrient consider-
ed, and here a figure of 50g protein per day has
been selected. This is based on the minimum physiological requirement, which for adults amounts to
30-35 g per day of an 'ideal' protein of perfect
quality that is wholly utilized by the body.
Proteins of most mixed diets are not perfect: they
have a quality rating (net protein utilization')
of 70, and thus 50 grams of food protein will provide 35 grams of 'ideal' or net-dietary protein.
The DHSS in fact recommend higher protein intakes
based on diets as conventionally eaten which provide
10 per cent of the energy as protein and which
at an intake of 2500 kcals would be about 60 grams
per day, but there is plenty of evidence that the
DHSS levels are unnecessarily high for the maintenance of nitrogen balance provided energy intake
is adequate.
      Of the minerals, only two were selected for
consideration, calcium and iron. Grain products

Table 14.2: The cost of nutrients as purchased in different foods in London in March 1965

Food	Price (d/1b)	Calories (d/2500 kcal)	Protein (d/50g)	Calcium (d/500 mg)	Iron (d/10mg)	Vitamin A (d/5000 i.u.)	Vitamin C (d/20mg)
Lard	13	8	*	*	*	*	*
Flour	6	10	6	6	8	*	*
Cooking fat	18	11	*	*	*	*	*
Oatmeal	9	12	8	18	5	*	*
Sugar	9	12	*	685	*	*	*
Margarine	18	13	20	469	125	7	*
Rice	11	17	20	313	53	*	*
Potatoes	3	19	16	43	9	*	0.7
Spaghetti	14	20	15	66	25	*	*
Bread	9	21	13	11	11	13	*
Butter	40	28	*	3125	*	*	*
Syrup	15	30	*	63	23	*	*
Cornflour	34	35	*	775	33	*	7.5
Jam	17	35	265	78	25	*	*
Cornflakes	25	38	41	370	19	*	*
Sausages	34	38	24	104	14	*	*
Peanuts	28	38	16	74	44	*	*
Haricot beans	18	38	9	11	6	*	*
Boiled sweets	24	40	*	535	125	*	*
Mutton	20	45	12	59	9	*	*
Toffees	36	45	190	42	52	30	*
Cheese	38	50	17	5	148	*	*
Bacon	36	55	27	274	75	*	*
Ham	54	58	39	422	99	*	*

Table 14.2: The cost of nutrients as purchased in different foods in London in March 1965 (contd.)

	Price (d/lb)	Calories (d/2500 kcal)	Protein (d/50g)	Calcium (d/500 mg)	Iron (d/10mg)	Vitamin A (d/5000 i.u.)	Vitamin C (d/20mg)
Brazil nuts	30	58	50	42	52	*	*
Milk chocolate	60	58	75	25	77	2970	*
Milk	9/pt	60	25	7	225	64	*
Herrings	24	73	21	34	44	225	*
Almonds	30	75	43	36	43	*	*
Gelatin	56	78	6	*	*	*	*
Eggs	33/doz	78	21	41	198	25	*
Apples	8	95	250	250	63	525	8
Sardines	55	103	30	15	304	605	8
Liver	34	130	23	442	5	2	*
Carrots	5	130	80	12	19	1	5.0
Cabbage	6	135	24	9	11	40	3.7
Bananas	12	145	190	335	107	200	0.5
Beef	48	150	27	1000	25	*	9
Pork	32	150	16	840	51	*	*
Chicken	18	170	17	660	107	*	*
Onions	8	178	85	28	56	*	*
Kippers	30	183	32	114	104	490	3.6
Pears	15	213	470	235	156	3000	*
Oranges	10	215	195	37	92	540	22
Beer	18/pt	250	640	145	*	*	1.2

Table 14.2: The cost of nutrients as purchased in different foods in London in March 1965 (contd.)

	Price (d/lb)	Calories (d/2500 kcal)	Protein (d/50g)	Calcium (d/500 mg)	Iron (d/10mg)	Vitamin A (d/5000 i.u.)	Vitamin C (d/20mg)
Cod	38	258	24	284	169	*	*
Frozen peas	36	308	70	258	42	24	0.6
Haddock	44	345	31	153	98	*	*
Pheasant	90	370	50	319	38	*	*
Tomatoes	10	390	100	82	53	29	2.2
Plaice	66	470	48	439	179	*	*
Salmon	152	663	140	915	649	845	*
Spinach	35	780	80	7	19	12	2.6
Whisky	534/bt	795	*	*	*	*	*
Watercress	24	938	90	12	33	16	1.7
Winkles	20/pt	1030	110	119	23	*	*
Frozen beans	46	1805	480	152	137	183	20
Mushrooms	48	3750	300	1880	104	*	*
Oysters	90/doz	6250	835	3310	250	2940	*

Note: All prices are shown in pre-decimal pence.
Cheapest foods are underlined.

are notoriously low in calcium which is therefore likely to be present in relatively small amounts in low-cost diets in the U.K. Although wheat is the staple foodstuff in Britain, compulsory fortification of flour with calcium carbonate offsets low intakes of calcium. Anaemia is common amongst women in Britain, especially during their menstrual years, and the regeneration of red blood cells is dependent upon an adequate source of iron. The DHSS recommended intakes of 500 mg per day of calcium and 10 mg of iron per day have been used.

Two vitamins were selected, retinol (vitamin A) and ascorbic acid (vitamin C), because they are particularly sensitive to cooking and processing losses. Also they occur in relatively expensive foods so that they are likely to be in short supply in low-cost diets. The FAO recommendation of 5000 i.u. of vitamin A per day and of 20 mg of vitamin C per day has been adopted. The B vitamins were considered only in the 1974 study, but were thought unlikely to be deficient in Britain where the staple food is wheat and moreover there is compulsory fortification of white flour with thiamin and nicotinic acid. There may be some nutritionists who would disagree with the recommended intakes chosen, but this is not important with respect of relative values of the foods as sources of nutrients.

The nutrient contents of the foods were calculated using standard food composition tables(2). These provide the concentration of nutrient per edible portion of food, from which the cost of providing the target quantity of each of the nutrients from each food could be calculated. For many of the items listed, such as flour, the cost of the 'as-purchased' material is the same as that for the 'edible portion'. However, in the case of fruit and vegetables, fish and meat, losses of the 'as-purchased' material occur as peelings and bones, and the cost of the 'edible portion' can be adjusted by the appropriate wastage factor given in the food tables. All the calculations for nutrients are for the raw foods. Cooking losses, particularly of the vitamins, are difficult to allow for as they vary with the severity and the method of cooking; the most conservative methods have been assumed.

Table 14.2 shows the cost of supplying the daily recommended intake of each of these nutrients by each food in the 1965 survey. Prices are given in old pence as this was before decimalization of money. The foods are listed in ascending order of cost to meet energy requirements. This is the prime factor in determining the adequacy of a diet and lack of calories presents the most important nutritional problem in the world today. Prices for the ten cheapest sources of each nutrient are underlined. These foods may be considered 'best buys' since they provide three or more nutrients at the cheapest rate. They include flour, oats, and potatoes, the staples of England, Scotland and Ireland; liver, carrots, and cabbage, very small amounts of which supply minerals and vitamins. Spinach, perhaps surprisingly, is not a particularly cheap source of iron. Watercress rates well, being a salad food, hence no cooking losses. Rice is demonstrably a less-useful cereal in this context than wheat-flour or oats. Mutton is the cheapest meat, providing cheaper protein than the cheapest fish, herring, which compares in price with egg. There are a number of anomalies in the table. Gelatine, although cheap, is a protein of little biological value, and would preferably be replaced by cheese or chicken. Mushrooms just provide flavour! Onions provide both flavour and cheap vitamin C, and interestingly cost the same for energy as chicken. Beer is second only to oysters for cost of protein, and not even very cheap for energy, whereas whisky provides expensive calories mainly due to tax.

All this is very entertaining, but is it useful? Such a table demonstrates very clearly that if one is constructing low-cost diets the major outlay is for calories and protein, and that foods of animal origin are the most expensive part of a diet. The vitamin and mineral requirements may easily be satisfied with a few pennyworth of liver, carrots and cabbage. This consideration could be important in giving advice to old-age pensioners and others with limited means. With these data it was calculated that in 1965 a person's nutrient needs could be obtained for one-shilling a day using a mixture of flour, lard, carrots and cabbage.

This exercise was repeated in 1974 and 1975, by which time the currency had changed. Table 14.3 shows prices in new pence per pound. It so happened that this also covered a period of rampant inflation. Most prices had at least doubled from 1965 to 1974 and many increased as much again from 1974 to 1975. From March 1965 to January 1974 food prices had increased at about 8.5 per cent per annum according to the retail food price index:

THE COST OF NUTRIENTS

Table 14.3: A survey of food prices in England, 1965-75

Food	Price (p/lb) 1965	Price (p/lb) 1974	Price (p/lb) 1975
Sugar	3.75	5.0	14.5
Flour	2.5	4.7	5.5
Lard	5.4	13.0	20.0
Butter	16.5	20.0	27.5
Margarine	7.5	15.0	20.0
Bread	3.75	6.5	7.5
Potatoes	1.2	3.0	4.0
Oatmeal	3.75	11.0	12.0
Rice	4.6	11.0	11.0
Spaghetti	4.7	14.0	19.0
Cornflakes	10.0	14.0	20.0
Cornflour	14.0	16.0	20.0
Milk (Pint)	3.75	5.5	6.0
Cheese	16.0	30.0	38.0
Eggs (1 doz standard)	14.0	40.0	34.0
Haricot beans	7.5	20.0	19.0
Bacon (Streaky)	15.0	35.0	58.0
Ham (Shoulder)	22.0	84.0	88.0
Mutton (Shoulder)	8.5	22.0	37.0
Sausages	14.0	23.0	28.0
Liver	14.0	36.0	38.0
Chicken	7.5	22.0	30.0
Beef (Stewing)	20.0	44.0	61.0
Carrots	2.0	3.0	8.0
Cabbage	2.5	6.0	10.0
Frozen spinach	15.0	12.0	18.0
Watercress	10.0	31.0	50.0
Frozen peas	15.0	13.0	17.5
Frozen beans	19.0	20.0	17.0
Onions	3.0	4.0	12.0
Cod fillet	16.0	52.0	60.0
Kippers	12.5	38.0	51.0
Oranges	4.5	10.0	14.0
Apples	2.3	6.0	15.0
Jam	7.0	12.0	21.0
Golden syrup	6.0	8.5	19.5
Tinned tomatoes	4.5	14.0	16.0
Mushrooms	20.0	24.0	32.0

Note: All prices expressed in new pence.

however, for the foods (except oysters) listed
in table 14.2 the inflation rate was 88 per cent,
equivalent to 9.8 per cent per annum, mostly of
course due to the higher inflation rates after
1970. From January 1974 to June 1975 the most
spectacular change was an increase of 190 per cent
for sugar; eggs, haricot beans and frozen beans
were slightly cheaper. The average price increase
for the 38 foods was about 50 per cent (33 per
cent per year), and this was for the cheapest buys.
Even the subsidized foods - flour and bread, milk,
and cheese - had doubled in price over the ten
years, and mutton had risen more dramatically than
beef.

In tables 14.4 to 14.9 foods are listed in
ascending order of cost for energy and the five
nutrients for each of the three years. Again the
'best buys' are underlined, that is foods proving
a cheap source of three or more nutrients in each
year. Cereals, potatoes, fats and sugar are consistently cheap sources of energy: indeed, nine
of the foods in table 14.4 are the same as those
named by Lusk in 1914. Cereals and potatoes are
also cheap protein sources (table 14.5) and it
is notable that haricot beans and peanuts
are strongly competitive with meat and dairy products. Dairy products, spinach and flour are the
cheapest sources of calcium (table 14.6); liver,
oatmeal, beans and flour (n.b. fortified) of iron
(table 14.7), but iron in liver is the most readily
absorbed by man. Liver and spinach again feature
prominently as sources of vitamin A (table 14.8).
It will be noted that the revised international
system for expressing recommended intakes of vitamin
A was adopted: 0.3 retinol-equivalents are equivalent to 1 i.u. vitamin A. Table 14.9 demonstrates
the advantages of modern food technology, whereby
frozen peas and spinach provide cheap vitamin C
throughout the year and a more reliable source
than cabbage and potatoes where long storage and
cooking times can deplete the vitamin C content.
In 1974 the cost of buying three vitamins of the
B group was calculated, viz. thiamin, riboflavin
and nicotinic acid, and cornflakes at 14p per lb
were by far the cheapest food, providing a day's
requirement for 3p, 3.5p and 3.5p respectively.
Beer was the most costly: it took 44 pints to provide the thiamin requirement!

In 1974 the cheapest cost for daily nutrients
including B vitamins came to 11p (compared with
5p in 1965). This was for a mixture of flour,

Table 14.4: Cheapest Energy Sources (pence/2500 kcals)

Rank	1965	(p/2500 kcals)	1974	(p/2500 kcals)	1975	(p/2500 kcals)
1	Lard	3.3	Sugar	7	Flour	8.8
2	Flour	4.2	Flour	7.5	Lard	12.2
3	Cooking fat	4.6	Lard	8	Margarine	14.0
4	Oatmeal	5.0	C. fat	9	Oatmeal	16.4
5	Sugar	5.0	Margarine	10.5	Rice	17.0
6	Margarine	5.5	Butter	14	Bread	17.3
7	Rice	7.1	Bread	15	Butter	19.3
8	Potatoes	8.0	Oatmeal	15	Sugar	20.5
9	Spaghetti	8.4	Syrup	16	Potatoes	25.3
10	Bread	8.8	Rice	17	Spaghetti	27.0
11	Butter	11.8	Potatoes	19	Cornflakes	30.0
12	Syrup	12.6	Spaghetti	20	Cornflour	31.3
13	Cornflour	15.5	Cornflakes	21	Syrup	37.0

Table 14.5: Cheapest Protein Sources (Pence/50g Protein)

Rank	1965	(p/50g)	1974	(p/50g)	1975	(p/50g)
1	Flour	2.5	Flour	5.0	Flour	5.9
2	Gelatin	2.5	Gelatin	6.5	Haricots	9.5
3	Oatmeal	3.4	Bread	9.2	Bread	10.6
4	Haricot beans	3.8	Peanuts	9.5	Oatmeal	10.9
5	Mutton*	5.0	Oatmeal	10.0	Milk	16.4
6	Bread	5.5	Haricot beans	10.0	Cheese	16.5
7	Spaghetti	6.3	Cheese	13.0	Rice	19.5
8	Potatoes	6.7	Mutton*	13.0	Sausages	19.5
9	Peanuts	6.7	Spaghetti	15.0	Spaghetti	20.4
10	Cheese	7.0	Milk	15.0	Eggs	21.3
11	Chicken	7.0	Potatoes	16.0	Potatoes	21.3
12	Rice	8.4	Herrings	17.5	Mutton*	21.8
13	Herrings	8.8	Rice	19.5	Liver	25.5

Note: * = shoulder

Table 14.6: Cheapest Calcium Sources(pence/500mg calcium) p/500mg (excluding the contribution from tap water)

Rank	1964	(p/500mg)	1974	(p/500mg)	1975	(p/500mg)
1	Cheese	2.1	Frozen Spinach	2.4	Frozen Spinach	3.6
2	Flour	2.5	Cheese	3.9	Milk	4.5
3	Milk	2.9	Milk	4.1	Cheese	5.0
4	Frozen Spinach	2.9	Flour	5.0	Flour	5.9
5	Cabbage	3.8	Carrots	7.0	Bread	9.2
6	Bread	4.6	Bread	8.0	Haricot beans	11.4
7	Haricot beans	4.6	Cabbage	9.0	Cabbage	15.0
8	Carrots	5.0	Onions	11.0	Carrots	18.7
9	Watercress	5.0	Haricot beans	12.0	Oatmeal	24.0
10	Sardines	6.3	Sardines	12.0	Watercress	24.2

Table 14.7: Cheapest Iron Sources (pence/10mg Iron)

Rank	1964	(p/10mg)	1974	(p/10mg)	1975	(p/10mg)
1	Liver	2.1	Liver	5.5	Liver	5.8
2	Oatmeal	2.1	Oatmeal	6.0	Haricot beans	6.2
3	Haricot beans	2.5	Flour	6.0	Oatmeal	6.5
4	Flour	3.4	Haricot beans	6.5	Flour	7.0
5	Potatoes	3.8	Frozen Spinach	6.5	Bread	9.2
6	Mutton	3.8	Bread	8.0	Frozen Spinach	9.8
7	Bread	4.6	Potatoes	9.0	Sausages	11.6
8	Cabbage	4.6	Sausages	9.5	Potatoes	12.0
9	Sausages	5.9	Mutton	10.0	Cornflakes	14.3
10	Frozen Spinach	8.0	Cornflakes	10.0	Mutton	16.8

THE COST OF NUTRIENTS

Table 14.8: Cheapest Sources of Vitamin A (pence/750mg Retinol-equivalents)

Rank	1964	(p/750mg)	1974	(p/750mg)	1975	(p/750mg)
1	Carrots	0.2	Carrots	0.3	Carrots	0.8
2	Liver	0.4	Liver	1.0	Liver	1.1
3	Margarine	1.5	Frozen Spinach	2.0	Frozen Spinach	3.0
4	Frozen Spinach	2.5	Watercress	2.2	Margarine	4.0
5	Butter	2.7	Margarine	3.0	Butter	5.5
6	Watercress	3.4	Butter	4.0	Frozen Peas	6.1
7	Frozen Peas	5.0	Frozen Peas	4.5	Eggs	12.8
8	Eggs	5.3	Cheese	12.0	Cheese	15.8
9	Tomatoes	6.1	Eggs	15.0	Watercress	17.0
10	Cheese	6.3	Tomatoes	20.0	Milk	21.8

Table 14.9: Cheapest Sources of Vitamin C (pence/20mg ascorbic acid)

Rank	1964	(p/20mg)	1974	(p/20mg)	1975	(p/20mg)
1	Cabbage	0.2	Frozen Peas	0.2	Frozen Peas	0.3
2	Frozen Peas	0.3	Cabbage	0.5	Cabbage	0.9
3	Potatoes	0.3	Potatoes	0.7	Potatoes	1.0
4	Oranges	0.5	Frozen Spinach	0.9	Frozen Spinach	1.4
5	Watercress	0.7	Oranges	1.2	Oranges	1.7
6	Tomatoes	0.9	Onions	1.8	Watercress	3.5
7	Frozen Spinach	1.1	Carrots	2.2	Tomatoes	3.5
8	Onions	1.5	Watercress	2.2	Onions	5.4
9	Carrots	1.6	Bananas	6.0	Carrots	5.9
10	Liver	2.1	Liver	6.0	Liver	6.0

liver, cornflakes, potatoes and margarine. However, in order to produce a palatable diet that would meet the criteria outlined at the beginning of this paper, expenditure in 1974 would have cost 25p per day, and in 1975 30-40p per day. In other words, this exercise strikingly demonstrates that at the very least 50 per cent and generally much more of food bills is spent on 'palatability' and the outlay for nutrients is but a small fraction of the total cost.

The data shown in tables 14.4 to 14.9 may suggest to historians that this would be a useful approach in looking at diets in history. If commodity prices are available, it is possible to work out with the aid of a set of food composition tables how cheaply people could live, and more importantly to judge the relative prices of commodities in terms of their nutrient contents. Of course people do not necessarily change their food habits to use new cheap sources of nutrients, but where food habits have changed one may be able to seek an explanation on the basis of changes in relative price of nutrients, particularly of energy, for example sugar.

A tentative application of this approach has been made using British retail prices from 1891-1938. Tables 14.10 and 14.11 set out the results, expressed as old pence per nutrient. It will be seen that as sources of energy the cheap buys are very familiar, and that there is little to choose between them until 1926, after which rice becomes more expensive relative to flour. The most expensive period was 1920, after which many food prices collapsed in the inter-war years: the cost of energy from sugar in 1920 was remarkably high at 16d, while mutton was as cheap a source of energy as cereals in 1938! In table 14.11 it is notable that potatoes provided cheap protein and were indeed on a par with flour in 1912-13. Finally, attention should be drawn to a feature about the dairy products, butter, milk and cheese not previously noted. In grouping these together it became apparent that the cost of nutrients from milk, the raw product, was greater than from cheese or butter - after the producer has made his profit selling milk to the cheese and butter factories, who in turn have to make their profit. It seems that the demand for milk was such that it could command a price in the market place that had no relationship whatsoever to its nutritional value. The same phenomenon still held good in 1965, but the situation had

Table 14.10: <u>The Relative Cost of Energy, 1890-1938</u> (old pence/2500 kcals)

Food	1891/2	1899/01	1912/13	1920	1926	1933	1936/7	1938
Flour	2	2	3	5	4	3	3	3
Oatmeal	3	2	3	-	4	4	6	4
Rice	3	3	3	-	4	5	6	7
Bread	3	3	3	7	5	4	5	4
Sugar	3	3	3	16	5	3	-	3
Potatoes	5	4	3	12	11	6	-	6
Lard	4	3	4	-	-	-	5	-
Margarine	-	-	5	9	8	4	-	5
Butter	11	9	10	24	14	9	11	11
Milk	18	11	12	30	23	19	-	22
Cheese	10	10	11	27	17	12	14	14
Mutton	8	6	5	7	8	4	11	4
Liver	-	19	15	-	-	8	34	38
Cabbage	-	39	22	-	-	22	28	22

Table 14.11: <u>The Relative Cost of Protein, 1890-1938 (old pence/50g protein)</u>

Food	1891/2	1899/01	1912/13	1920	1926	1933	1936/7	1938
Flour	1	1	2	3	3	2	2	2
Oatmeal	2	1	2	-	3	3	4	3
Rice	3	4	4	-	4	5	7	8
Bread	2	2	2	4	3	3	3	3
Potatoes	4	3	2	10	9	5	-	5
Milk	8	5	5	13	10	8	-	9
Cheese	3	3	4	9	6	4	5	5
Mutton	6	5	4	6	6	3	9	3
Liver	-	3	3	-	-	1	6	7
Cabbage	-	7	4	-	-	4	5	4

changed by 1974-5, when cheese had become more expensive although butter was still a cheaper source of energy.

Inevitably, the early data from the 1890s to 1930s raise some interesting questions. It would appear that during this period man could live on 5d per day - which invites further study of consumption in relation to wage rates. The cheapness of mutton is outstanding - which contrasts with known levels of consumption of this meat. The relationship of relative prices to the patterns of consumption during this period remain to be explored more fully.

NOTES

1. D.S. Miller and P. Mumford, 'Scrooge in the Kitchen', Getting the Most out of Food, (1966) No. 2, p. 9; R. Wilson, 'An investigation into low-cost dietaries' M.Sc. Thesis, 1974, University of London; G. Chapman and P. Mumford, 'Economy and Palatability', Nutrition and Food Science 43 (1976), p. 10.
2. A.A. Paul and D.A.T. Southgate, The Composition of Foods M.R.C, S.R. No. 297 (1978).

15. THE FOUNDING FATHERS OF THE NUTRITION SOCIETY(1)

ALICE M. COPPING

Of the eleven leading nutritionists who signed the original circular inviting interest in forming an official Nutrition Society in 1941, ten were men who were already heavily involved in the national war effort and one was a woman, Dr. (later Dame) Harriette Chick (1875-1977) who may well be called the mother of nutrition in this country. All were distinguished in their widely diverse fields but were of like mind in that they cared deeply for the health and welfare of the nation and indeed of other nations as well.

Sir John Orr (1880-1971), later Lord Boyd Orr, was the prime mover in encouraging the extension of the informal meetings that had been organized by Dr. S.K. Kon of the National Institute for Research in Dairying into a full Nutrition Society. Orr was trained both in agriculture and in medicine and was Director of the Rowett Research Institute at Aberdeen. In addition he carried much advisory responsibility to government departments concerned with production and distribution of food for man and animals. He was particularly well qualified to realize the need for a meeting place for all concerned with food and nutrition. His dynamic personality and his almost uncanny gifts of persuasion are well illustrated in his calling together the preliminary meetings at the Royal Institution to discuss the founding of the Nutrition Society and then arranging the initial committee with members most likely to get things moving rapidly even amid the exigencies of wartime. In 1941 he was already crossing the Atlantic by convoy or by air to discuss a World Food Plan, with a view to post-war reconstruction. This was an optimistic view not universally shared but one which Orr himself pursued firmly until the Hot

Springs Conference was called in 1943 to be followed in 1945 by the Quebec meeting and the establishment of the first international agency of the United Nations - the Food and Agriculture Organization. Not surprisingly, in the face of his magnificent address to the Quebec Conference, Orr was invited to become the first Director General of the Food and Agriculture Organization (FAO). Although he was already 65 and had decided to retire from public life and give more time to his Angus farm and to his parliamentary duties, Orr decided to accept the challenge and to take the post for two years in order to set the new organization on its way. He began by providing himself with a knowledgeable nucleus staff with international experience of food supplies and food needs. A hasty survey of the world food position led to a special meeting of all governments in 1946 to consider urgent food problems. At that time the FAO under its existing constitution had not effective powers to deal with the ominous food situation but an International Emergency Food Council was set up to be paid for by FAO and to promote as quickly as possible an international allocation of major foodstuffs that were in short supply. The work of the new Council encouraged Orr to make a new attempt to persuade governments to change the constitution of FAO and to provide the organization with sufficient funds and authority to engage through a World Food Board in a larger and more significant enterprise. In spite of further conferences this was never fully implemented but Orr's foundation activities in FAO gave it the grand start that has led to its world-wide involvement with food production and use. After he retired from FAO in 1948 Orr continued to travel the world as a representative of world peace and other international movements. In 1949 he was awarded the Nobel Peace Prize. He was known and honoured the world over and wherever he went the impact of his forthright and practical personality stirred enthusiasm for his aims. He was a tall spare Scot with astonishing eyebrows above clear blue eyes, an inspiration to work for and a joy to meet on unexpected occasions. His fine energy faltered a little at the end of his long life but in his 91st year his mind was still clear and his memory good.

In 1931, just ten years before the founding of the Nutrition Society, Sir John Orr and Sir Charles Martin (1866-1955) were jointly concerned in the publication of the first volume of Nutrition

<u>Abstracts and Reviews</u>, which was planned to provide
a service for nutritionists and medical and agricultural research workers and field workers who could
not make easy contact with libraries and other
sources of information. For its first 30 years
<u>Nutrition Abstracts and Reviews</u> was edited jointly
from the Rowett Institute in Aberdeen and the Lister
Institute in London, where Dr. Chick took up editorial duties from Sir Charles Martin on his retirement to an advisory post in Australia. Martin
returned to England in 1933 and settled in Cambridge
where he continued his interest in nutrition studies
and provided a working place for the Division of
Nutrition of the Lister Institute when it had to
be removed from the Chelsea building on the outbreak
of war in 1939. He was thus firmly involved in
the plans for the Nutrition Society and presided
over the first general meeting in October 1941
when Orr was called away to an urgent conference
in the USA. Martin was already 75 in 1941 but
his interest and enthusiasm were undiminished.
Shortly after obtaining his qualification in medicine in 1891 Martin went to Australia as demonstrat-
or in physiology in the newly formed Medical School
of the University of Sydney. There he instituted
classical research into the action of snake venom
which earned him fellowship of the Royal Society
in 1901. After six years in Sydney he transferred
to Melbourne where he became Professor of Physiology and inspired many young students to work in
widely different fields of research and subsequently
to become directors of research around the world.
In 1903 Martin was called back to London to be
Director of the Lister Institute but his 12 years
in Australia had implanted a great enjoyment of
outdoor activities that continued throughout his
life and brought him friends and colleagues who
kept contact and visited him whenever they came
to London or Cambridge. He was interested in animal
nutrition as well as human problems and his work
and advice in both fields was eminently practical.
He was very generous in giving his ideas, his time
and his energy to any research or to such a project
as the Nutrition Society which pleased his active
mind.

Dr. Harriette Chick came to the Lister Institute in 1905 and fell immediately under the spell
of Martin who subsequently inspired her to change
her field of research from problems of bacteriology
to those of nutrition, arising from his service
with the Medical Corps of the Australian Army in

the Middle East in 1915. The wartime studies prepared her for leading the team of five women who
went to Vienna in 1919 on behalf of the Lister
Institute and the Medical Research Committee (later
the Medical Research Council) to investigate the
relation of nutrition to rickets and osteomalacia.
On her return to London in 1922 her work at the
Lister Institute continued in research on proteins,
vitamins of the B complex including the role of
maize in causing pellagra and the nutritive value
of other cereals. The outbreak of war in 1939
found her at retiring age but quite undeterred
in energy and ideas, so that her Division of Nutrition happily found a wartime home in Martin's house
beside the Cam at Old Chesterton in Cambridge.
There the Division attended to its research, took
care of the food production in the large garden
and helped actively with the preliminary planning
for the Nutrition Society. Her interest and participation in meetings of the Society continued
into her 100th year and she lived half way into
her 103rd year. Orr lived to 91, Martin to 89,
so these three founders were a good indication
of the longevity of nutritionists.

Sir Frederick Gowland Hopkins (1861-1947)
was 80 when he supported the Nutrition Society
at its foundation and indeed gave the opening address at its inaugural meeting in October 1941.
In his long years as Professor of Biochemistry
in Cambridge he was not only the father of British
biochemistry but also a massive contributor to
thought and experiment in the biochemical field
throughout the world. His early nutritional studies
established the existence of accessory food factors,
later to be termed vitamins, and he carried his
ideas on biochemistry and nutrition into ingenious
experimental work that had much practical application for animals and man. He had met and formed
a lasting friendship with Charles Martin when they
were pre-medical students in London and their contact continued through the years of retirement
when neither relinquished his interest in vital
research and advancement of science. Hopkins was
a small and gentle man but with a tremendous personal power of inspiring others to work and carry
out new ideas. He did not expect his students
or his colleagues to carry on research in the lines
that interested him at any one time but rather
helped them to expand and express their own ideas,
so he was a most excellent guide and philosopher
in the biochemical world until he left us at the

320

age of 86.

Sir Edward Mellanby (1884-1955) was Secretary of the Medical Research Council (MRC) and his name on the foundation circular gave his blessing not only to the new Nutrition Society but at the same time encouraged the participation of members of the staff of Medical Research Council Institutes, notably those of the Dunn Nutritional Institute in Cambridge without whose efforts none of the highly demanding secretarial and organizational work could have been initiated. Mellanby had a long history of nutrition research in the field of fat-soluble vitamins A and D beginning before the first world war and continuing into his time of appointment as Secretary of the Medical Research Council. His fundamental work on rickets in puppies was related to the efficacy of cod liver oil and butterfat in preventing experimental rickets and gave indications for the later separation of vitamins A and D in oils. He also showed the role of vitamin A in bone development and in his position as Secretary of the MRC fostered much nutrition research.

Professor J.C. (late Sir Jack) Drummond (1891-1952) was another live-wire biochemical nutritionist, who in 1941 was Scientific Adviser to the Ministry of Food and most anxious for a meeting place for all concerned with food and health. His own interests in biochemistry and nutrition were extra-ordinarily diverse and he had a great talent for imparting enthusiasm to others. He was appointed to teach physiological chemistry in the pre-medical faculty at University College London in 1919 and became the first occupant of the chair of biochemistry there when it was founded in 1922. His researches there were mainly on fats and fat-soluble vitamins, but at the same time he maintained interest in proteins and water-soluble vitamins. Some of the early work on the nature of the vitamin B complex came from his department which expanded rapidly and became an important centre for the growing subject of biochemistry in the 1920s. Nutrition as a practical application of biochemical studies became a paramount interest in Drummond's life and he studied the history of the subject as well as its current phases. He was admirably suited to his wartime post with the Ministry of Food and a considerable asset to the activities of the Nutrition Society, so his untimely death in 1952 caused dismay to all his friends and colleagues.

Sir Joseph Barcroft (1872-1947) had retired as Professor of Physiology in Cambridge in 1937 and become Director of the Unit of Animal Physiology of the Agricultural Research Council. He was also chairman of the Food Investigation Board, so he had many reasons for interest in and encouragement of the Nutrition Society. From the outset he gave the new society unstinted and unfailing service until the eve of his sudden death in 1947, when the loss of his benevolent presence and influence as President in succession to Sir John Orr was indeed grievous. The fact that he was 75 seemed surprising since he was so active mentally and physically. He was to be found in his office early and late and business was never delayed by any lack of communication. His unvarying good humour and infinite grace in dealing with all sorts of people was a great help to the Nutrition Society in its original plans and in the problems of achieving publication of its Proceedings under wartime exigencies of paper shortage and finance. Somehow he always knew the right place to look for help and his powerful persuasion obtained it. This applied especially in the matter of planning and carrying out the meeting of European nutritionists in the United Kingdom in 1946, with the eventual result of the institution of the International Congress of Nutrition which now meets worldwide. He came from a Quaker family in County Down and retained their high ideals and simple ways throughout his life. He so obviously enjoyed all that he undertook that it was a pleasure to work with him and a great boost for a new society. He had great gifts of presiding over discussions and making excellent summaries of a day of diverse papers, as illustrated by his masterly concluding remarks that ended some of the early meetings and still make good reading in the Proceedings.

Another distinguished Cambridge physiologist, Dr. (later Sir) John Hammond (1889-1964) brought a strong practical mind into the Nutrition Society. His concern with research in animal physiology and reproduction had built him a world reputation in animal breeding and meat production. He had extensive contact with many countries overseas both before and after the war and when the time came for expansion of the Nutrition Society his help in the office of President from 1947 to 1950 was most important, but right from the beginning his knowledge of the field of animal nutrition was a great asset in planning meetings and attracting the interest of workers in animal research and industry. He too had a gift for dealing with people and an ease of manner that made communication simple.

Dr. Leslie Harris (1898-1973), Director of the Dunn Nutritional Laboratory, not only signed the original circular but put a great deal of his own time and energy and also that of members of his staff into the project of establishing the Nutrition Society. He was the first secretary and gave a shining example for future secretaries in his way of dealing with correspondence and finding extensive voluntary aid for the society. His truly inspired appointment of Dr. Ethel Cruickshank as Minutes Secretary for the first Committee Meeting gave the Society a recorder for its first 30 years, so that the bound volumes of Committee and Council Minutes preserve accurately and fully the whole story of its growth and development. Dr. Harris was responsible for much of the detailed work of arranging the first international meeting, that of European nutritionists in 1946. He put very great effort into assuring further international cooperation and getting the International Union of Nutritional Sciences (IUNS) recognized as a member of the International Council of Scientific Unions. This was achieved only in 1968, although the healthy existence of IUNS had by then been well proven by seven most successful congresses in different countries. Through these meetings many new nutrition societies were inaugurated so that IUNS is now a flourishing concern bearing witness to the foresight of Dr. Harris and to his interest in spreading nutritional ideas abroad.

Professor H.D. Kay (1893-1977), Director of the National Institute for Research in Dairying, in signing the original circular brought into the foundation of the Nutrition Society the very solid cooperation of the staff of his institute in a way that has persisted throughout the whole history of the 48 years of the Society. Kay himself was a biochemist who had worked with Drummond at University College before he took the chair of biochemistry at the University of Toronto in Canada, whence he returned to Shinfield as Director of the Institute of Research in Dairying. There his wide knowledge of biochemistry and his great talent for encouraging research and ability in gaining personal cooperation made him a considerable power in the field of dairy technology. He was well aware of the need for nutritionists from different areas of the subject to meet for discussion and he gave active encouragement to Dr. Kon in the organization of the informal meetings of nutritionists that were held during the first 18 months of the war. With the establishment of the official Society again he gave the help of his staff needed in various capacities. As soon as the publication of Proceedings became possible Dr. Kon was selected as Editor and held the editorial chair until 1965. During all those years the Institute provided accommodation and much other assistance in the publications of the Nutrition Society. Dr. Kay kept up his own interest in the Society up to and beyond his retirement, when he continued to be involved in matters concerned with food, nutrition and health to the end of his long life. His friendly presence at meetings continued until he died in 1977 at the age of 84, when he still looked and seemed almost as young as at the time of his retirement many years earlier.

Sir Rudolph Peters (1889-1982), who died recently in his nineties, was Professor of Biochemistry at Oxford at the time of the foundation of the Nutrition Society. His laboratory made great contributions to research in nutritional biochemistry and many of his colleagues have served the Nutrition Society during the years. On retirement he went to live in Cambridge and kept up a lively interest in research and in the Nutrition Society. He had been a student of Sir Frederick Hopkins and had taught in the Biochemistry Department in Cambridge before being appointed to the Oxford chair which he held from 1923 to 1954. His continued presence at meetings gave further testimony of the longevity of nutritionists. None of the original signatories died before the age of 75, except Sir Jack Drummond, and most were many years beyond that age.

In the inaugural discussions on founding the Society Sir John Orr very wisely suggested that as travel was difficult during the war there should be a Scottish group with some independence. Professor R.C. Garry was asked to organize the Scottish Branch and he called a meeting at the University of Dundee in January 1942 to set up their first committee. Full liaison between English and Scottish Groups was established and maintained during the war and in 1945, when hostilities had ceased the general adjustment of affairs was in progress, the Scottish Group expressed their wish to remain an autonomous group and not to become